Contents

- Coconut Cream Pie 4
- The Great Pumpkin Pie 5
- Savory Tomato Galette 7
- Crunchy Caramel Apple Pie 8
- Zesty Lemon Squares 9
- Red Velvet Whoopie Pies 10
- S'mores Cookies 11
- The Softest Peanut Butter Cookies 12
- Dunkable Chocolate Chip Cookies 13
- Thin Mint Copycat Cookies 14
- Blackberry Shortbread Thumbprints 15
- Easy Frosted Sugar Cookies 16
- Snickerdoodle Apple Cobbler 18
- Sliced Banana Bread Cobbler 19
- Easy Blackberry Cobbler 20
- The Easiest Baked Flatbread 20
- Garlic and Herb Focaccia 21
- Thin and Crispy Pizza Crust 22
- Skillet Pizza Crust 23
- Coconut Macaroons 25
- Cranberry Oatmeal Cookies 26
- Sensational Snickerdoodles 26
- Biscotti 27
- Decadent Chocolate Cobbler 29
- Pear Pecan Crisp 30
- Classic Cheesecake 31
- Triple-Layer Birthday Cake with Buttercream Frosting 32
- Chocolate Crack Pie 33
- Perfect Piecrust 34
- Blueberry Crumble Slab Pie 35
- Cinnamon Roll Pancakes 37
- The Infamous Pumpkin Muffins 38
- Double-Chocolate Chunk Muffins 39
- Sweet Blackberry Muffins 40
- Oatmeal Blueberry Muffins 41
- Thin Mint Cupcakes 42

Very Strawberry Cupcakes	43
Fudgy Chocolate Cupcakes	44
Samoa Donuts	46
Delicious Donut Holes	48
Italian Zeppoli (Sfingi)	48
Cannoli	49
Pepperoni Pizza Rolls	51
Stromboli Pockets	52
Sicilian Deep-Dish Pizza	54
Everything Bagels	55
Soft Pretzels	57
Skillet Cherry Cobbler	58
Very Berry Cobbler	59
Peach Cobbler	61
Vanilla Cupcakes	62
Pumpkin Pie Cupcakes	63
Gingerbread Cupcakes	64
Death-by-Chocolate Cake	65
Super Moist Cream Cheese Pound Cake	66
Buttery Mini Tarts	67
Vanilla Donuts	69
Beignets	70
Apple Cider Cinnamon Donuts	71
Garlic Butter Breadsticks	73
Perfect Skillet Pancakes	75
Mom's French Toast	75
Overnight Waffles	76
Glazed Lemon Poppy Seed Loaf	77
Cinnamon Swirl Loaf	78
Double-Chocolate Zucchini Bread	79
Chocolate Chip Banana Bread	80
Apple Cinnamon Muffins	81
Coffee Cake Muffins	82
Veggie Muffins	83
Easy Drop Biscuits	84
Garlic and Herb Drop Biscuits	85
Classic Biscuits	86
Toasted Coconut Apple Raspberry Crisp	88

Strawberry Streusel Crisp	89
Angel Food Cake	90
Carrot Cake	91
Gooey Butter Cake	92
Lemon Lover's Bundt Cake	93
Lemon Crème Brûlée Pie	95
Éclair Pie	96
Baked Apple Cinnamon Hand Pies	97
Sweet Tart Cakelets	98
Italian Cream Tarts (Pasticciotti)	99
Cinnamon Rolls	101
Strawberry Shortcake Rolls	103
Lemon Berry Turnovers	105
PB&J Turnovers	106
Mini French Crullers	107
Butterhorns	108
Cream Puffs	109
Homemade Graham Crackers	110
Pastry Dough	111
Choux Pastry	112
Sandwich Bread	113
Burger Buns	114
Artisan Loaves	115
Soft French Loaves	116
Pillowy Dinner Rolls	117
Tortilla Wraps	118

Coconut Cream Pie

MAKES 1 (9-INCH) PIE

Prep time: 1 hour 25 minutes, plus 3 hours to chill

Cook time: 27 minutes

Ingredients:

- 200 grams shredded coconut, divided
- Shortening, for preparing the pie plate
- 1 single Perfect Piecrust
- 4 large egg yolks
- 1 teaspoon vanilla extract
- 125 grams All-Purpose Flour Blend
- ¼ teaspoon xanthan gum
- ¼ teaspoon salt
- 1 (14-ounce) can coconut cream
- 1 cup cold whole milk or coconut milk beverage
- 133 grams cane sugar or granulated sugar
- 2 tablespoons butter or nondairy alternative
- Whipped cream or nondairy alternative, for serving

Directions:

Step 1

Preheat the oven to 325°F. Line a baking sheet with parchment paper.

Step 2

Spread 100 grams of coconut into a thin layer on the prepared baking sheet. Bake for 5 to 7 minutes, or until golden. Set the coconut aside until serving time.

Step 3

Coat a 9-inch pie plate with shortening and fit the piecrust into the pie plate. Shape the edges to your liking. Refrigerate for 1 hour.

Step 4

Preheat the oven to 400°F.

Step 5

Line the piecrust with parchment or aluminum foil (shiny-side down) and fill the bottom with dried beans or pie weights. Blind bake the crust for about 15 minutes, or until the edges are golden. Remove from the oven and remove the lining and weights. Prick holes all over the bottom of the crust with a fork. Return to the oven for 10 to 12 minutes, until the crust begins to brown. Let it cool completely as you prepare the filling.

Step 6

In a medium bowl, whisk the egg yolks and vanilla. In a small bowl, whisk together the flour, xanthan gum, and salt.

Step 7

In a large saucepan, whisk the coconut cream, milk, and sugar together over medium heat. Bring it to a boil, whisking occasionally, for about 2 minutes, then remove from the heat.

Step 8

Whisk the flour mixture into the egg mixture. Then, whisking constantly, use a ladle to slowly add a small and steady stream of the warm cream mixture to the flour/egg mixture. Keep whisking so the egg yolks do not scramble. Repeat with one more ladle of cream mixture.

Step 9

Return the saucepan to low heat and combine all of the mixture into it. Bring to a simmer for 3 to 4 minutes, or until the mixture is bubbling and thickened slightly.

Step 10

Remove the saucepan from the heat and stir in the butter and remaining 100 grams of coconut.

Step 11

Pour the filling into the baked piecrust and cover it tightly with plastic (the plastic should be touching the filling). Chill the pie for at least 3 hours or overnight for best results.

Step 12

Serve the pie topped with whipped cream and sprinkled with the toasted coconut. This pie is best served cold. Refrigerate leftovers, covered, for up to 3 days.

The Great Pumpkin Pie

MAKES 1 (9-INCH) PIE

Prep time: 30 minutes

Cook time: about 1 hour 10 minutes

Ingredients:

FOR THE PIECRUST

- Shortening, for preparing the pie plate
- 1 double Perfect Piecrust

FOR THE FILLING

- 20 grams All-Purpose Flour Blend
- 2 teaspoons ground cinnamon
- ½ teaspoon salt
- ¼ teaspoon ground nutmeg
- ¼ teaspoon ground cloves
- ¼ teaspoon xanthan gum
- Sprinkle freshly ground black pepper
- 4 large eggs, divided
- 1 (**Step 7**4-ounce) can sweetened condensed coconut milk
- ¼ cup maple syrup
- 1 (15-ounce) can pumpkin puree

FOR THE COCONUT WHIPPED CREAM

- 1 (14-ounce) can coconut cream, refrigerated overnight
- 2 tablespoons powdered sugar

Directions:

TO MAKE THE PIECRUST

Step 1

Preheat the oven to 425°F. Lightly grease a 9-inch pie plate with shortening. Line a baking sheet with parchment paper.

Step 2

Prepare the dough and roll out one portion as directed. Fit the dough round into the pie plate as directed and crimp the edges.

Step 3

Roll out the second portion and place it on the prepared baking sheet. Refrigerate both crusts while you make the filling.

TO MAKE THE FILLING

Step 4

In a small bowl, whisk the flour, cinnamon, salt, nutmeg, cloves, xanthan gum, and pepper to combine.

Step 5

In a large bowl, whisk 3 of the eggs and the condensed milk until smooth and creamy with zero lumps. Using a spatula, stir in the maple syrup until combined. (I do not recommend using a handheld electric mixer for this step.) Add the flour mixture and pumpkin and stir again just until combined with no lumps, stopping to scrape the edges of the bowl, as needed. Do not overmix.

Step 6

Remove the bottom crust in the pie plate from the refrigerator and pour the filling into it.

Step 7

In a small bowl, whisk the remaining egg and 1 tablespoon water to create an egg wash. Using a pastry brush, lightly brush the edges of the crust with the egg wash. Reserve the remaining egg wash.

Step 8

Bake for 10 minutes, then (without opening the oven) reduce the oven temperature to 350°F and bake for 30 to 35 minutes more, or until the center is set. Turn off the oven, crack open the oven door, and leave the pie in the oven for 10 to 15 minutes to adjust to the change in temperature.

Step 9

Transfer the pie to a wire rack and let it cool completely, at least 2 to 3 hours, before serving.

Step 10

While the pie cools, preheat the oven to 350°F. Line a baking sheet with parchment paper.

Step 11

Remove the second portion of rolled-out dough from the refrigerator. Using cookie cutters, make leaf or pumpkin shapes to decorate the pie. If the dough is too hard, let it sit a few minutes. Transfer the shapes to the clean prepared baking sheet and lightly brush them with the remaining egg wash.

Step 12

Bake for 10 minutes, or until golden.

Step 13

Let the shapes cool on the baking sheet for at least 10 minutes, then gently transfer to a wire rack to cool completely.

TO MAKE THE COCONUT WHIPPED CREAM

Step 14

Open the chilled can of coconut cream and pour off the watery liquid. Scoop only the solid part into a large bowl and add the powdered sugar. Using a handheld electric mixer, beat until smooth and fluffy.

Step 15

Place the cooled cutouts on top of the cooled pie. Slice and serve with a dollop of coconut whipped cream.

Step 16

Refrigerate leftover pie and whipped cream separately, covered, for up to 3 days.

Savory Tomato Galette

MAKES 1 (9-INCH) GALETTE

Prep time: 1 hour 30 minutes

Cook time: about 1 hour

Ingredients:

- All-Purpose Flour Blend, for dusting
- 1 double Perfect Piecrust
- 1½ pounds heirloom tomatoes, thinly sliced
- 2 garlic cloves, minced
- 1 teaspoon salt
- ½ teaspoon freshly ground black pepper
- 60 grams Gouda or cheddar cheese or nondairy alternative, grated
- 1 tablespoon grated Parmesan cheese or nondairy alternative
- 4 fresh basil leaves, halved
- 1 large egg
- 1 teaspoon dried oregano
- ½ teaspoon red pepper flakes

Directions:

Step 1

Line a baking sheet with parchment paper. Dust a work surface with flour. Weigh out 500 grams of the pie dough, about two-thirds of the full recipe (save the rest for kids' treats; see Tip). Roll the dough into a round about 12 inches across and a little more than ⅛ inch thick. Transfer the dough to the prepared baking sheet and refrigerate for at least 1 hour.

Step 2

Preheat the oven to 400°F. Line a baking sheet with aluminum foil. Line a large plate with paper towels.

Step 3

Arrange the tomato slices in a single layer on the prepared baking sheet and sprinkle with the garlic, salt, and pepper.

Step 4

Bake for 5 minutes. The tomatoes will start releasing some juice. Drain off the juice and transfer the tomatoes to the paper towels.

Step 5

Remove the dough from the refrigerator and let sit for a minute to soften. Sprinkle the Gouda and Parmesan over the dough, leaving a clean 1½-inch border all around. Place the tomatoes over the cheese. Arrange the basil evenly on top. Bring the edges of the dough up and over the filling, overlapping pieces, as needed, to create a border that is 1½ inches wide.

Step 6

In a small bowl, whisk the egg and 1 tablespoon water to create an egg wash. Using a pastry brush, brush the egg wash over the border.

Step 7

Freeze the galette for 10 minutes.

Step 8

Bake for 55 to 60 minutes, or until the crust is golden brown.

Step 9

Let the galette cool slightly. Sprinkle with the oregano and red pepper flakes. Serve warm. Refrigerate leftovers in an airtight container for up to 3 days.

Crunchy Caramel Apple Pie

MAKES 1 (9-INCH) PIE

Prep time: 45 minutes

Cook time: 55 minutes

Ingredients:

FOR THE PIECRUST

- Shortening, for preparing the pan
- 1 single Perfect Piecrust

FOR THE FILLING

- 100 grams cane sugar or granulated sugar
- 32 grams All-Purpose Flour Blend
- 1 teaspoon ground cinnamon
- ¼ teaspoon xanthan gum
- ¼ teaspoon salt
- 720 grams very thinly sliced peeled Honeycrisp or Granny Smith apples

FOR THE CRUMBLE TOPPING AND DRIZZLE

- 200 grams light brown sugar
- 62 grams All-Purpose Flour Blend
- 50 grams certified gluten-free rolled oats
- ¼ teaspoon xanthan gum
- 8 tablespoons (1 stick) cold butter or nondairy alternative
- 31 grams chopped pecans
- ¼ cup salted caramel sauce (from <u>Salted Caramel Brownies</u>)

Directions:

TO MAKE THE PIECRUST

Step 1

Preheat the oven to 375°F. Lightly grease a 9-inch pie plate with shortening.

Step 2

Roll out and fit the piecrust into the prepared plate as directed and refrigerate it.

TO MAKE THE FILLING

Step 3

In a large bowl, whisk the cane sugar, flour, cinnamon, xanthan gum, and salt to combine. Using a spatula, fold in the apples, covering them completely in the flour mixture.

Step 4

Remove the piecrust from the refrigerator and pour the apple mixture into it. Return it to the refrigerator.

TO MAKE THE CRUMBLE TOPPING

Step 5

In a medium bowl, whisk the brown sugar, flour, oats, and xanthan gum to combine. Cut the butter into pieces and add it to the oat mixture. Using a pastry cutter, cut the butter into the oats until coarse crumbs form.

Step 6

Remove the filled crust from the refrigerator and cover it evenly with the crumble topping. Loosely cover the edges of the crust with aluminum foil.

Step 7

Bake for 25 minutes. Remove the foil and bake for 25 to 30 minutes more, or until the filling is bubbling and the crust is golden.

Step 8

Transfer to a wire rack to cool.

TO FINISH THE PIE

Step 9

Sprinkle the pie with pecans and drizzle the salted caramel sauce over the top. Refrigerate leftovers, covered, for up to 3 days.

Zesty Lemon Squares

MAKES 9 SQUARES

Prep time: 25 minutes
Cook time: 45 minutes

Ingredients:

FOR THE CRUST

- 190 grams All-Purpose Flour Blend
- ½ teaspoon xanthan gum
- ½ teaspoon salt
- 12 tablespoons (1½ sticks) butter or nondairy alternative, melted and slightly cooled
- 100 grams cane sugar or granulated sugar
- 1 teaspoon vanilla extract

FOR THE FILLING

- 2 large eggs
- 200 grams cane sugar or granulated sugar
- 62 grams All-Purpose Flour Blend
- ½ teaspoon baking powder
- ¼ teaspoon xanthan gum
- ¼ teaspoon salt
- 1 tablespoon grated lemon zest (about 1 large lemon)
- ½ cup fresh lemon juice (about 3 large lemons)
- 3 tablespoons powdered sugar

Directions:

TO MAKE THE CRUST

Step 1

Preheat the oven to 350°F. Line a 9-by-9-inch baking pan with parchment paper, leaving some hanging over the edges. This will make the bars easy to remove.

Step 2

In a medium bowl, whisk the flour, xanthan gum, and salt to combine. Using a spatula, stir in the melted butter, sugar, and vanilla. Pour the crust into the prepared baking pan and spread it evenly.

Step 3

Bake for 20 minutes. Remove and leave the oven on.

TO MAKE THE FILLING

Step 4

While the crust bakes, in a small bowl, using a handheld electric mixer, beat the eggs.

Step 5

In a medium bowl, whisk the sugar, flour, baking powder, xanthan gum, and salt to combine. Add the beaten eggs, lemon zest, and lemon juice and mix well.

Step 6

Pour the filling evenly over the crust, then return to the oven and bake for 20 to 25 minutes, or until the middle is set and does not jiggle.

Step 7

Let the bars cool for 10 to 20 minutes, then cover with aluminum foil and refrigerate at least 1 hour.

Step 8

Dust the squares with the powdered sugar before serving. Refrigerate the bars, covered, for up to 5 days.

Red Velvet Whoopie Pies

MAKES 14 SANDWICH COOKIES

Prep time: 2 hours 35 minutes

Cook time: 12 minutes

Ingredients:

FOR THE PIES

- 250 grams All-Purpose Flour Blend
- 15 grams unsweetened natural cocoa powder
- 1 teaspoon baking soda
- ½ teaspoon xanthan gum
- ½ teaspoon salt
- 8 tablespoons (1 stick) butter or nondairy alternative
- 200 grams light brown sugar
- 1 large egg
- ⅔ cup whole milk or coconut milk beverage
- 2 teaspoons vanilla extract
- ½ teaspoon apple cider vinegar
- 1 teaspoon red gel food coloring

FOR THE FILLING

- 51 grams shortening
- 4 ounces cream cheese or nondairy alternative
- 1 tablespoon whole milk or coconut milk beverage
- 1 teaspoon vanilla extract
- 300 grams powdered sugar

Directions:
TO MAKE THE PIES
Step 1

In a medium bowl, whisk the flour, cocoa powder, baking soda, xanthan gum, and salt to combine.

Step 2

In a large bowl, using a handheld electric mixer on medium speed, cream the butter. Add the brown sugar and mix until well combined. Add the egg and mix well again. Add the milk, vanilla, and vinegar and mix again. The mixture will look curdled. That's okay.

Step 3

Add half the flour mixture and mix to combine. Add the remaining flour mixture and mix again. Add the red food coloring and mix until completely incorporated.

Step 4

Refrigerate for 2 hours to set, until the mixture looks like thick cupcake batter. During the last few minutes of chilling, preheat the oven to 350°F and line 2 baking sheets with parchment paper. (Don't use silicone mats because they might stain.)

Step 5

Using a 1-inch ice cream scoop, transfer tablespoon-size mounds of the batter onto the prepared baking sheets about 3 inches apart.

Step 6

Bake for 10 to 12 minutes until the centers appear set but the cookies are still soft. Cool for 10 minutes on the baking sheets, then gently transfer to a wire rack to cool completely.

TO MAKE THE FILLING
Step 7

In a medium bowl, using a handheld electric mixer on medium speed, cream together the shortening and cream cheese until smooth and creamy. Add the milk and vanilla. Mix, then add the powdered sugar and mix well until smooth.

Step 8

Pair the red velvet cookies by size. Spread a generous layer of filling on the inside of one cookie and top it with the other to form a sandwich. Repeat with the remaining cookies.

Step 9

Keep in an airtight container at room temperature for up to 3 days, or refrigerate for up to 5 days.

S'mores Cookies

MAKES 12 COOKIES
Prep time: 30 minutes
Cook time: 18 minutes per batch

Ingredients:
- 50 grams mini marshmallows
- 250 grams All-Purpose Flour Blend
- 52 grams finely crushed <u>Homemade Graham Crackers</u> or gluten-free graham cracker crumbs
- 2 teaspoons arrowroot
- 1 teaspoon baking soda
- ½ teaspoon xanthan gum

- ½ teaspoon salt
- 8 tablespoons (1 stick) butter or nondairy alternative
- 150 grams light brown sugar
- 50 grams cane sugar or granulated sugar
- 1 large egg
- 2 teaspoons vanilla extract
- 180 grams semisweet chocolate chips or nondairy alternative

Directions:

Step 1

Preheat the oven to 375°F. Line 2 baking sheets with parchment paper or silicone baking mats.

Step 2

Cut the mini marshmallows in half using kitchen shears.

Step 3

In a medium bowl, whisk the flour, graham cracker crumbs, arrowroot, baking soda, xanthan gum, and salt to combine.

Step 4

In a large bowl, using a handheld electric mixer on medium speed, cream together the butter, brown sugar, and cane sugar. Add the egg and vanilla. Mix well to combine. Beat in the flour mixture in two additions and mix to form a dough. Using a spatula, fold in half the marshmallows and half the chocolate chips. The batter will be thick and sticky.

Step 5

Using tablespoon-size portions, roll the dough into balls and place them on the prepared baking sheets 3 inches apart.

Step 6

Bake one batch at a time. Transfer to the oven and bake for 8 minutes. The cookies will still be very soft. Remove from the oven and top each cookie with some of the remaining marshmallows and chocolate chips.

Step 7

Return to the oven and bake for 7 to 10 minutes more, or until the cookies are golden on the edges and soft in the middle.

Step 8

Let the cookies cool on the baking sheet for 10 minutes, then gently transfer them to a wire rack to cool completely.

Step 9

Keep the cookies in an airtight container at room temperature for up to 5 days or freeze for up to 1 month.

The Softest Peanut Butter Cookies

MAKES 24 COOKIES

Prep time: 1 hour 15 minutes
Cook time: 12 minutes per batch

Ingredients:

- 156 grams All-Purpose Flour Blend
- ½ teaspoon baking soda
- ½ teaspoon xanthan gum

- 8 tablespoons (1 stick) butter or nondairy alternative
- 100 grams light brown sugar
- 50 grams cane sugar or granulated sugar, plus 2 tablespoons
- 180 grams creamy gluten-free peanut butter
- 1 large egg
- 1 teaspoon vanilla extract

Directions:

Step 1

In a small bowl, whisk the flour, baking soda, and xanthan gum to combine.

Step 2

In a large bowl, using a handheld electric mixer on medium speed, cream together the butter, brown sugar, and 50 grams of cane sugar. Add the peanut butter and mix until smooth and creamy. Add the egg and vanilla. Mix until combined.

Step 3

Slowly add the flour mixture and mix until combined. Do not overmix. Cover the bowl with plastic wrap and refrigerate for at least 1 hour.

Step 4

Preheat the oven to 350°F. Line 2 baking sheets with parchment paper or silicone baking mats.

Step 5

Place the remaining 2 tablespoons of cane sugar in a small bowl.

Step 6

Using a 1-inch ice cream scoop, scoop the cookies and gently roll them in the cane sugar to coat lightly. Place the cookies on the prepared baking sheets 3 inches apart. Using the tines of a fork, make a crisscross imprint on each one.

Step 7

Baking one batch at a time, bake for 10 to 12 minutes, or until the edges are slightly browned. The cookies will still be very soft and may have small cracks.

Step 8

Let the cookies cool on the baking sheet to continue baking without becoming overdone. Gently transfer to a wire rack. Keep in an airtight container at room temperature for up to 7 days.

Dunkable Chocolate Chip Cookies

MAKES 34 COOKIES

Prep time: 45 minutes

Cook time: 12 minutes per batch

Ingredients:

- 210 grams All-Purpose Flour Blend
- 1 teaspoon baking soda
- ½ teaspoon xanthan gum
- ½ teaspoon salt
- 51 grams shortening
- 133 grams light brown sugar
- 1 large egg

- 2 tablespoons maple syrup
- 2 teaspoons vanilla extract
- ½ teaspoon apple cider vinegar
- 225 grams semisweet chocolate chips or nondairy alternative

Directions:

Step 1

Line 2 baking sheets with parchment paper or silicone baking mats.

Step 2

In a small bowl, whisk the flour, baking soda, xanthan gum, and salt to combine.

Step 3

In a medium bowl, using a handheld electric mixer on medium speed, cream together the shortening and brown sugar. Add the egg, maple syrup, vanilla, and apple cider vinegar. Mix again until combined. Add the flour mixture and mix to form a dough. Using a spatula, fold in the chocolate chips.

Step 4

Using a 1-inch ice cream scoop, scoop the cookies onto one of the prepared baking sheets. It's okay if they are close together. Refrigerate for 30 minutes.

Step 5

Preheat the oven to 375°F.

Step 6

Transfer half of the chilled cookies onto the second prepared baking sheet, placing them 3 inches apart. Leave the remaining cookies in the refrigerator.

Step 7

Bake the first batch for 10 to 12 minutes, or until lightly browned on the sides.

Step 8

Let the cookies cool on the baking sheet for 10 minutes, then transfer to a wire rack to cool completely.

Step 9

Refill the baking sheet with the chilled cookies from the fridge and bake as directed.

Thin Mint Copycat Cookies

MAKES 28 COOKIES

Prep time: 15 minutes, plus 30 minutes to chill
Cook time: 10 minutes per batch

Ingredients:

FOR THE COOKIES

- 190 grams All-Purpose Flour Blend
- 75 grams Dutch-process cocoa powder
- 1 teaspoon baking powder
- ½ teaspoon xanthan gum
- ¼ teaspoon salt
- 179 grams shortening
- 200 grams cane sugar or granulated sugar
- 1 large egg
- 1 teaspoon vanilla extract

- ¼ teaspoon peppermint extract

FOR THE COATING

- 360 grams semisweet chocolate chips or nondairy alternative
- ½ teaspoon coconut oil, melted
- ¼ teaspoon peppermint extract

Directions:

TO MAKE THE COOKIES

Step 1

Preheat the oven to 350°F. Line 2 baking sheets with parchment paper. Cut two additional large sheets of parchment for rolling the dough.

Step 2

In a medium bowl, whisk the flour, cocoa powder, baking powder, xanthan gum, and salt to combine.

Step 3

In a large bowl, using a handheld electric mixer on medium speed, cream together the shortening and sugar, stopping to scrape down the bowl as needed. Add the egg, vanilla, and peppermint extract and mix until combined. Add the flour mixture and mix until combined. The dough will look slightly sticky.

Step 4

Transfer the dough to one sheet of parchment paper and place the other on top. Roll the dough to a large round about ¼ inch thick. Using a 2-inch round cookie cutter, cut out the cookies and place them on the baking sheets. Reroll the remaining dough and repeat until no dough is left.

Step 5

Baking one sheet at a time, bake for 8 to 10 minutes.

Step 6

Let the cookies cool on the pan for 10 minutes, then transfer to a wire rack. They will be soft at first but will crisp as they cool.

TO MAKE THE COATING

Step 7

In a medium saucepan, melt the chocolate over medium-low heat, stirring constantly so it does not burn. Stir in the coconut oil and peppermint extract.

Step 8

Dip each cookie in the melted chocolate and coat completely. Using a fork, lift them out of the chocolate, letting any excess fall back into the pan. Place the dipped cookies back on the parchment-lined baking sheets. Refrigerate for 30 minutes to help the chocolate set.

Step 9

Just like traditional Thin Mints, these cookies are best eaten cold. Refrigerate leftovers in an airtight container for up to 1 week or freeze for up to 1 month.

Blackberry Shortbread Thumbprints

MAKES 24 COOKIES

Prep time: 20 minutes, plus 30 minutes to chill
Cook time: 14 minutes per batch

Ingredients:

- 250 grams All-Purpose Flour Blend

- 1 teaspoon xanthan gum
- ½ teaspoon baking powder
- 136 grams shortening
- 133 grams cane sugar or granulated sugar
- 1 teaspoon vanilla extract
- ½ teaspoon orange extract
- ½ cup blackberry jam
- Glaze (from Cinnamon Roll Pancakes)

Directions:

Step 1

Line 2 baking sheets with parchment paper or silicone baking mats.

Step 2

In a small bowl, whisk the flour, xanthan gum, and baking powder to combine.

Step 3

In a large bowl, using a handheld electric mixer on medium speed, cream together the shortening and sugar. Add the vanilla and orange extract and mix to combine. Add flour mixture and mix to form a dough.

Step 4

Using 1-tablespoon portions, roll the dough into balls and place them on the prepared baking sheets. Gently make a thumbprint in the center of each cookie. Smooth any cracks along the outer edges with your fingers. Fill each thumbprint with about ½ teaspoon of jam. Refrigerate for 30 minutes.

Step 5

Preheat the oven to 350°F.

Step 6

Baking one batch at a time, bake for 12 to 14 minutes, or until the edges are slightly browned.

Step 7

Let the cookies cool on the pan for 5 to 10 minutes, then gently transfer to a wire rack to cool completely.

Step 8

Using a fork, drizzle the glaze over the cookies. Let set and dry for about 1 hour. Keep in an airtight container at room temperature for up to 5 days, or freeze for up to 1 month.

Easy Frosted Sugar Cookies

MAKES 16 COOKIES

Prep time: 1 hour 20 minutes

Cook time: 13 minutes per batch

Ingredients:

FOR THE COOKIES

312 grams All-Purpose Flour Blend, plus more for dusting

½ teaspoon xanthan gum

½ teaspoon baking powder

¼ teaspoon salt

102 grams shortening

150 grams cane sugar or granulated sugar

1 large egg

2 teaspoons vanilla extract

¼ teaspoon orange extract

¼ cup plus 1 tablespoon cold water

FOR THE FROSTING

240 grams powdered sugar

¼ cup whole milk or coconut milk beverage

½ teaspoon vanilla extract

Directions:

TO MAKE THE COOKIES

Step 1

In a small bowl, whisk the flour, xanthan gum, baking powder, and salt to combine.

Step 2

In a large bowl, using a handheld electric mixer on medium speed, cream together the shortening and sugar. Add the egg, vanilla, and orange extract and mix to combine. Slowly add the flour mixture and cold water. Stir until coarse crumbs form. Continue to form the dough by hand. The warmth of your hands will help the dough come together.

Step 3

Divide the dough into 4 equal portions, wrap each in plastic wrap, and chill for 30 minutes to 1 hour. Any longer and your dough will be too hard to work with and you will need to let it sit on the counter for 5 to 10 minutes so it is easier to work with.

Step 4

Preheat the oven to 350°F. Line 2 baking sheets with parchment paper or silicone baking mats.

Step 5

Place two sheets of parchment paper on a work surface and dust them with flour. Place one dough portion between the two sheets of parchment and roll it to ¼-inch thickness. Using cookie cutters, cut the dough into desired shapes and transfer them to the prepared baking sheets. Gather the scraps and repeat the steps with the remaining 3 dough portions.

Step 6

Bake for 11 to 13 minutes. The cookies will be soft but very lightly browned around the edges.

Step 7

Let the cookies cool on the baking sheet for 10 minutes, then use a spatula to gently transfer them to a wire rack to cool completely.

TO MAKE THE FROSTING

Step 8

In a medium bowl, stir together the powdered sugar, milk, and vanilla until smooth.

Step 9

Dip each cookie top into the icing, then transfer to a wire rack. Allow the icing to set for about 1 hour.

Step 10

Keep the cookies in an airtight container at room temperature for up to 4 days. They can be frozen without icing for up to 1 month in a freezer bag. Separating the cookies with parchment paper before freezing helps keep them fresh.

Snickerdoodle Apple Cobbler

MAKES 1 (9-BY-13-INCH) COBBLER

Prep time: 30 minutes

Cook time: 35 minutes

Ingredients:

- Shortening, for preparing the pan

FOR THE SNICKERDOODLE TOPPING

- 190 grams All-Purpose Flour Blend
- 150 grams cane sugar or granulated sugar
- 1 teaspoon xanthan gum
- 1 teaspoon cream of tartar
- 1 teaspoon ground cinnamon
- ½ teaspoon baking soda
- ½ teaspoon salt
- 8 tablespoons (1 stick) butter or nondairy alternative
- 1 large egg

FOR THE CINNAMON SUGAR

- 2 tablespoons cane sugar or granulated sugar
- 1 teaspoon ground cinnamon

FOR THE FILLING

- 100 grams cane sugar or granulated sugar
- 32 grams All-Purpose Flour Blend
- ¼ teaspoon xanthan gum
- 1 teaspoon ground cinnamon
- 1,200 grams sliced peeled Granny Smith or Honeycrisp apples
- 1 tablespoon fresh lemon juice
- 1 teaspoon vanilla extract

Directions:

Step 1

Preheat the oven to 375°F. Grease a 9-by-13-inch pan with shortening.

TO MAKE THE SNICKERDOODLE TOPPING

Step 2

In a medium bowl, whisk the flour, sugar, xanthan gum, cream of tartar, cinnamon, baking soda, and salt to combine.

Step 3

Cut the butter into pieces and add it to the flour mixture along with the egg. Using a handheld electric mixer, mix the ingredients. The dough may seem dry and crumbly, but that is okay. Set aside.

TO MAKE THE CINNAMON SUGAR

Step 4

In a small bowl, stir together the sugar and cinnamon.

TO MAKE THE FILLING

Step 5

In a large bowl, whisk the sugar, flour, xanthan gum, and cinnamon to combine. Add the apples and, using a spatula, fold them into the flour mixture. Sprinkle the lemon juice and vanilla over the top and give it all another stir.

Step 6

Pour the apples evenly into the prepared pan. Using your clean hands, flatten pieces of snickerdoodle topping and place them over the apples as close together as possible to form a crust. Sprinkle the cinnamon sugar over the top.

Step 7

Bake for 20 minutes. Check that it is not browning too quickly. Loosely cover with aluminum foil, if needed, and bake for 15 minutes, or until the top is golden and the apples are bubbling.

Step 8

Serve warm. Refrigerate leftovers, covered, for up to 3 days. Reheat to serve.

Sliced Banana Bread Cobbler

MAKES 1 (9-BY-9-INCH) COBBLER
Prep time: 30 minutes
Cook time: 40 minutes

Ingredients:

- Shortening, for preparing the pan
- 200 grams light brown sugar
- 32 grams All-Purpose Flour Blend
- ½ teaspoon ground cinnamon, plus more for sprinkling
- ¼ teaspoon xanthan gum
- 5 bananas, sliced
- 1 large egg, beaten
- 1 cup whole milk or coconut milk beverage
- 8 tablespoons (1 stick) butter or nondairy alternative, melted
- 6 or 7 slices Chocolate Chip Banana Bread , made without the chocolate chips

Directions:

Step 1

Preheat the oven to 350°F. Grease a 9-by-9-inch pan with shortening.

Step 2

In a large bowl, whisk the brown sugar, flour, cinnamon, and xanthan gum to combine. Add the bananas and stir to coat them well. Spread the bananas in the prepared pan. The pan should be about half full. Add or subtract pieces, if needed.

Step 3

In a small bowl, whisk the egg, milk, and melted butter until blended.

Step 4

Cut the crusts off the bread if desired, then cut each slice into thin strips. Lay the bread strips over the bananas.

Step 5

Pour the egg mixture over the top. Do not stir. Sprinkle lightly with cinnamon.

Step 6

Bake for 35 to 40 minutes, or until golden.

Step 7

Refrigerate leftovers in an airtight container for up to 3 days.

Easy Blackberry Cobbler

MAKES 1 (9-BY-13-INCH) COBBLER

Prep time: 10 minutes
Cook time: about 1 hour

Ingredients:

- Shortening, for preparing the pan
- 250 grams cane sugar or granulated sugar, divided
- 125 grams All-Purpose Flour Blend
- 1½ teaspoons baking powder
- ½ teaspoon xanthan gum
- ½ teaspoon salt
- 1 cup whole milk or coconut milk beverage
- 4 tablespoons butter or nondairy alternative, melted
- ½ teaspoon apple cider vinegar
- 230 grams blackberries
- 2 tablespoons raw turbinado sugar

Directions:

Step 1

Preheat the oven to 350°F. Grease a 9-by-13-inch baking dish with shortening.

Step 2

In a medium bowl, whisk 200 grams of cane sugar, the flour, baking powder, xanthan gum, and salt to combine. Using a spatula, stir in the milk, melted butter, and vinegar, mixing just until combined.

Step 3

Pour the batter into the prepared baking dish. Arrange the blackberries on top so they are evenly distributed. They will sink into the dough as they bake. Sprinkle the remaining 50 grams of cane sugar over the blackberries.

Step 4

Bake for 50 minutes. Remove and sprinkle the turbinado sugar over the top. Return to the oven and bake for 10 minutes more, or until golden brown. Serve warm.

Step 5

Refrigerate leftover cobbler, covered, for up to 3 days. Reheat to serve.

The Easiest Baked Flatbread

MAKES 1 (10-INCH) FLATBREAD

Prep time: 15 minutes
Cook time: 25 minutes

Ingredients:

- 62 grams Bread Flour Blend, plus more for dusting

- 2 teaspoons baking powder
- ½ teaspoon xanthan gum
- 120 grams plain Greek yogurt or nondairy alternative
- 1 tablespoon extra-virgin olive oil

Directions:

Step 1

Position an oven rack in the lower third of the oven. Place a cast-iron skillet or baking sheet in the oven to preheat, and set the oven to 375°F.

Step 2

Place a sheet of parchment paper on a work surface and lightly dust it with flour.

Step 3

In a medium bowl, whisk the flour, baking powder, and xanthan gum to combine. Using a wooden spoon or spatula, stir in the yogurt until a smooth dough ball forms.

Step 4

Transfer the dough to the floured parchment. Pour the olive oil into a small bowl. Dip your fingertips in the oil and flatten the dough into a 10-inch round about ¼ inch thick. Do not use a rolling pin. If the dough sticks to your fingertips, lightly dip them in the oil again. Lightly brush the remaining oil over the top of the flatbread.

Step 5

Trim the parchment paper so there is plenty of border around the flatbread and it will fit in the skillet. Using the parchment, transfer the flatbread to the preheated skillet or baking sheet.

Step 6

Bake for 10 minutes. Using a fork, lift one edge of the flatbread and remove the parchment. Bake directly in the pan or on the baking sheet for 10 to 15 minutes more, or until crisp. This is best served the same day.

Garlic and Herb Focaccia

MAKES 1 (9-INCH) FOCACCIA

Prep time: 2 hours 15 minutes
Cook time: 22 minutes

Ingredients:

- 8 tablespoons olive oil, divided, plus more for the baking dish and your fingertips
- 282 grams Bread Flour Blend
- 2 teaspoons xanthan gum
- 1 teaspoon baking powder
- 1½ teaspoons salt
- ¼ teaspoon garlic powder
- 2 teaspoons cane sugar or granulated sugar
- 1 (7-gram) packet instant (fast-acting) yeast
- 1 cup warm (100° to 110°F) water
- 2 garlic cloves, minced
- Fresh or dried herbs of choice, for topping
- Coarse sea salt
- Freshly ground black pepper

Directions:

Step 1

Lightly grease a 9-inch round glass baking dish with oil.

Step 2

In a medium bowl, whisk the flour, xanthan gum, baking powder, salt, and garlic powder to combine.

Step 3

In a large bowl, stir together the sugar, yeast, and warm water. Let stand for 5 minutes.

Step 4

Add 3 tablespoons of the oil and stir again. Using a handheld electric mixer fitted with the dough hook, add half the flour mixture to the yeast mixture, and mix on low speed to combine. Add the remaining flour and mix until a dough forms.

Step 5

Coat your fingertips in oil and transfer the dough to the prepared baking dish, spreading it evenly and folding down the edges. Cover tightly with plastic wrap and let rise for 1 hour, or until almost doubled in size.

Step 6

Using a spatula, gently lift each side of the bread while pouring 3 tablespoons of oil underneath the dough. Slide the dough around in the baking dish to distribute the oil. Re-cover the pan tightly with plastic and refrigerate for at least 1 hour.

Step 7

Preheat the oven to 450°F. Let the hot oven sit empty for at least 15 minutes at full temperature before baking.

Step 8

In a small bowl, whisk the remaining 2 tablespoons of oil, the garlic, and herbs to taste until blended. Season with salt and pepper and whisk to combine.

Step 9

Using your fingers, create dimples all over the surface of the dough. Using a pastry brush, brush the herb oil over the dough.

Step 10

Bake for 20 to 25 minutes, or until golden. If desired, broil the focaccia for 1 to 2 minutes to give it extra color and toast the garlic.

Step 11

Let the focaccia cool in the dish for 10 minutes before slicing and serving warm, or transfer to a wire rack to cool completely. Keep leftovers covered at room temperature for up to 2 days, or refrigerate for up to 1 week. Rewarm to serve.

Thin and Crispy Pizza Crust

MAKES 2 (10-INCH) CRUSTS

Prep time: 1 hour 20 minutes
Cook time: 25 minutes

Ingredients:

- 375 grams All-Purpose Flour Blend , plus more for dusting
- 2 tablespoons xanthan gum

- 1½ teaspoons salt
- 1 (7-gram) packet instant (fast-acting) yeast
- 1 tablespoon cane sugar or granulated sugar
- 1 cup (100° to 110°F) warm water
- ¼ cup olive oil, plus 1 tablespoon
- 1 large egg, beaten
- 1 tablespoon honey
- ½ teaspoon apple cider vinegar
- Pizza sauce, for topping
- Toppings of choice

Directions:

Step 1
Position an oven rack in the lower third of the oven. Place two sheets of parchment paper on a work surface and dust with flour.

Step 2
In a medium bowl, whisk the flour, xanthan gum, and salt to combine.

Step 3
In a large bowl, stir together the yeast, sugar, and warm water. Let sit for 5 minutes.

Step 4
Stir in ¼ cup of oil, the beaten egg, honey, and vinegar. Using a handheld electric mixer fitted with the dough attachment, add half the flour mixture and mix on low speed to combine. Add the remaining flour mixture and mix to form a dough.

Step 5
Pour the remaining 1 tablespoon of oil into a small bowl. Dip your fingertips in the oil and transfer the dough to the floured parchment. Divide the dough into 2 portions. (If only using one crust, see Tip.)

Step 6
Roll one portion of dough between the two sheets of parchment to about ⅛ inch thick. Use your hands to adjust the edges and create a nice round. Transfer the dough on the parchment to a pizza pan. If making a second crust, pull out another sheet of parchment paper and dust it with flour, then repeat the rolling process. Let the pizza round(s) rest and rise for at least 1 hour.

Step 7
Preheat the oven to 450°F.

Step 8
Bake one pizza crust for 5 minutes. Remove the crust from the oven and slide the parchment out from underneath, leaving the crust on the pan. Top as desired with sauce, cheese, and other toppings of choice. Bake for 15 to 20 minutes more, or until crisp. Repeat for a second pizza if making one.

Step 9
Let the pizza sit for 5 minutes before slicing. Refrigerate leftovers, covered, for up to 3 days.

Skillet Pizza Crust

MAKES 2 (12-INCH) CRUSTS
Prep time: 1 hour 50 minutes
Cook time: 25 minutes

Ingredients:

- 375 grams <u>All-Purpose Flour Blend</u> , plus more for dusting
- 1 tablespoon xanthan gum
- 1½ teaspoons salt
- 1 (7-gram) packet instant (fast-acting) yeast
- ¼ cup olive oil, plus 2 tablespoons
- 1 large egg
- 1 tablespoon honey
- 1½ cups plus 2 tablespoons warm (100° to 110°F) water
- Pizza toppings, of choice

Directions:

Step 1

Position an oven rack in the lower third of the oven.

Step 2

Cut a piece of parchment paper to 14 inches. Fold it into fourths and round off the corners. Open the parchment into a round. Repeat to make one more parchment round.

Step 3

Place an additional piece of parchment on a work surface. Place one round on top and dust it with flour.

Step 4

In a medium bowl, whisk the flour, xanthan gum, salt, and yeast to combine.

Step 5

In a large bowl, using a handheld electric mixer, beat ¼ cup of oil, the egg, and honey, mixing until the egg is fully beaten. Add the warm water and mix for 1 minute. Add the flour mixture and mix until combined and a wet dough forms; it will look like batter. Using a spatula, fold the dough into a ball.

Step 6

Pour the remaining 2 tablespoons of oil into a small bowl. Coat your fingers and palms in about 1 tablespoon of the oil and swipe the edge of a bench scraper with oil as well. Using the bench scraper, cut down the middle of the dough and lift one half, transferring it to the flour-dusted parchment round.

Step 7

Using oiled hands, spread the dough from the middle outward into a 12-inch round. If the dough sticks to your fingers, dab them with more oil. Be careful not to flood the dough with too much oil. Slide the crust to the side using the parchment round.

Step 8

Place the second parchment round on your work surface and dust it with flour. Transfer the remaining dough to the parchment round and repeat step 7 with the remaining 1 tablespoon of oil. (If not baking 2 pizzas, shape and refrigerate the second crust for the next day.)

Step 9

Let the dough rest for 1 to 1½ hours.

Step 10

Preheat the oven to 425°F. Preheat a cast-iron skillet in the hot oven for at least 30 minutes.

Step 11

Transfer one crust, on the parchment round, to a pizza peel or rimless baking sheet and carefully slide the crust, still on the parchment, into the hot skillet.

Step 12

Bake for 5 minutes.

Step 13

Using oven mitts, remove the skillet from the oven and place it on a heat-resistant surface. Using the bench scraper, lift one edge of the crust and gently grab the parchment and remove it.

Step 14

Add any desired toppings to the pizza. Bake for 20 to 25 minutes more, or until the outer crust is golden and crisp.

Step 15

Remove from the oven, lift one edge of the pizza with a utensil, and slide it onto a tray or plate. Let the pizza cool for a few minutes before slicing and serving.

Step 16

If making the second pizza, repeat to bake and top as directed.

Coconut Macaroons

MAKES 18 MACAROONS

Prep time: 45 minutes
Cook time: 15 minutes per batch

Ingredients:

- 42 grams All-Purpose Flour Blend
- ¼ teaspoon xanthan gum
- ¼ teaspoon salt
- 1 (**Step 7**4-ounce) can sweetened condensed coconut milk
- ½ teaspoon orange extract or almond extract
- 1 teaspoon vanilla extract
- 1 large egg white, beaten
- 100 grams unsweetened coconut flakes

Directions:

Step 1

In a small bowl, whisk the flour, xanthan gum, and salt to combine.

Step 2

In a medium bowl, whisk the condensed milk and extracts. Add the beaten egg white and whisk to combine. Stir in the flour mixture and coconut flakes, mixing well. Cover the bowl with plastic wrap and refrigerate for 30 minutes.

Step 3

Preheat the oven to 350°F. Line 2 baking sheets with parchment paper or silicone baking mats.

Step 4

Using a 1-inch ice cream scoop, scoop the macaroons onto the prepared baking sheets. Smooth the bottom edges.

Step 5

Baking one batch at a time, bake for 12 to 15 minutes, or until the coconut looks slightly toasted.

Step 6

Let the cookies cool on the pan for at least 10 minutes, then gently transfer to a wire rack to cool completely. Keep covered and at room temperature for up to 5 days.

Cranberry Oatmeal Cookies

MAKES 24 COOKIES

Prep time: 15 minutes
Cook time: 10 minutes per batch

Ingredients:

- 300 grams certified gluten-free rolled oats
- 156 grams All-Purpose Flour Blend
- 1 teaspoon baking soda
- 1 teaspoon ground cinnamon
- ¼ teaspoon ground nutmeg
- ¼ teaspoon xanthan gum
- ¼ teaspoon salt
- 16 tablespoons (2 sticks) butter or nondairy alternative
- 200 grams light brown sugar
- 2 large eggs
- 1 teaspoon vanilla extract
- 150 grams dried cranberries

Directions:

Step 1

Preheat the oven to 350°F. Line 2 baking sheets with parchment paper or silicone baking mats.

Step 2

In a food processor, pulse the oats 5 or 6 times to break them down.

Step 3

In a medium bowl, whisk the flour, baking soda, cinnamon, nutmeg, xanthan gum, and salt to combine. Whisk in the oats and set aside.

Step 4

In a large bowl, using a handheld electric mixer on medium speed, cream together the butter and brown sugar. Add the eggs and vanilla. Mix well to combine. Beat in the flour mixture in two additions and mix to form the dough. Using a spatula, fold in the cranberries.

Step 5

Using tablespoon-size portions, roll the dough into balls and place them on the prepared baking sheets 3 inches apart.

Step 6

Baking one batch at a time, bake for 10 minutes, or until the edges are crispy.

Step 7

Let cookies cool on the baking sheets for 10 minutes, then gently transfer them to a wire rack to cool completely. Keep in an airtight container at room temperature for up to 5 days.

Sensational Snickerdoodles

MAKES 24 COOKIES

Prep time: 1 hour 15 minutes
Cook time: 13 minutes per batch

Ingredients:

- 190 grams All-Purpose Flour Blend
- 1 teaspoon xanthan gum
- 1 teaspoon cream of tartar
- 2 teaspoons ground cinnamon, divided
- ½ teaspoon baking soda
- ½ teaspoon salt
- 8 tablespoons (1 stick) butter or nondairy alternative
- 2 ounces cream cheese or nondairy alternative
- 150 grams cane sugar or granulated sugar, plus 2 tablespoons
- 1 large egg
- 2 teaspoons vanilla extract

Directions:

Step 1

In a small bowl, whisk the flour, xanthan gum, cream of tartar, 1 teaspoon of cinnamon, the baking soda, and salt to combine.

Step 2

In a large bowl, using a handheld electric mixer on medium speed, cream together the butter and cream cheese until smooth. Mix in 150 grams of sugar until well combined. Add the egg and vanilla and mix to combine, stopping to scrape down the bowl as needed.

Step 3

Beat the flour mixture into the cream cheese mixture in two additions, mixing to form a dough. This dough will be thick and pasty. Transfer the dough to an airtight container and refrigerate for at least 1 hour, or overnight for best results.

Step 4

Preheat the oven to 350°F. Line 2 baking sheets with parchment paper. (I recommend parchment because these cookies are so soft that the silicone mats will grip the edges but leave a hollow middle.)

Step 5

In a small bowl, stir together the remaining 1 teaspoon of cinnamon and the remaining 2 tablespoons of sugar.

Step 6

Using tablespoon-size portions, roll the chilled dough into balls. Roll the balls in the cinnamon sugar and place them on the prepared baking sheet 3 inches apart. Fill both baking sheets. While one sheet is in the oven, place the other in the refrigerator.

Step 7

Bake for 11 to 13 minutes, or until the edges are set. The cookies will still be soft. Do not overbake.

Step 8

Let the cookies cool completely on the baking sheet, where they will continue baking without becoming overdone. Bake the second batch as directed. Keep in an airtight container at room temperature for up to 5 days.

Biscotti

MAKES 16 BISCOTTI
Prep time: 15 minutes

Cook time: 45 minutes

Ingredients:

- 190 grams All-Purpose Flour Blend
- 60 grams brown rice flour
- 1 teaspoon baking powder
- ½ teaspoon xanthan gum
- ½ teaspoon salt
- 4 tablespoons butter or nondairy alternative
- 150 grams cane sugar or granulated sugar
- 3 large eggs, divided
- 1½ teaspoons vanilla extract
- ½ teaspoon orange extract

Directions:

Step 1

Preheat the oven to 350°F. Line 2 baking sheets with parchment paper or silicone baking mats.

Step 2

In a medium bowl, whisk the all-purpose flour, brown rice flour, baking powder, xanthan gum, and salt to combine.

Step 3

In a large bowl, using a handheld electric mixer on medium speed, cream together the butter and sugar. Add 2 of the eggs and the vanilla and orange extracts, and mix until combined. Add the flour mixture and mix until combined, stopping to scrape down the bowl as needed. Your dough will resemble a very thick batter.

Step 4

Add about 1 tablespoon of water to a piping bag and rub the bag from the outside to spread the water inside the bag. This will help the dough slide through the bag. Fill the piping bag with the biscotti dough. Cut the tip of the bag a little bit bigger than 1 inch wide. Squeeze the dough into two equal-size logs onto one baking sheet. With wet fingertips, flatten the logs until they are about 1 inch in height.

Step 5

In a small bowl, whisk the remaining egg and 1 tablespoon water to create an egg wash. Using a pastry brush, lightly brush the egg wash over the top of each log.

Step 6

Bake for 20 to 25 minutes. Remove from the oven, but leave the oven on.

Step 7

Let the logs cool on the baking sheet for at least 30 minutes.

Step 8

With a sharp nonserrated knife, cut each log on the diagonal into ¾-inch-thick slices. Push down on the knife rather than saw, to prevent the cookies from breaking. Place each cookie on the second prepared baking sheet, cut-side up.

Step 9

Return to the oven and bake for 12 to 14 minutes, or until golden, with crisp edges.

Step 10

Let the biscotti cool on the pan for about 10 minutes, then transfer to a wire rack to cool completely. They will continue to crisp as they cool. Keep in an airtight container at room temperature for 1 to 2 weeks or freeze for up to 3 months.

Decadent Chocolate Cobbler

MAKES 1 (9-BY-9-INCH) COBBLER

Prep time: 15 minutes
Cook time: 30 minutes

Ingredients:

FOR THE COBBLER

- Shortening, for preparing the pan
- 125 grams All-Purpose Flour Blend
- 1 tablespoon arrowroot
- 2 teaspoons baking powder
- 1½ tablespoons Dutch-process cocoa powder
- ½ teaspoon salt
- ¼ teaspoon xanthan gum
- 133 grams cane sugar or granulated sugar
- ½ cup whole milk or coconut milk beverage
- 2 tablespoons butter or nondairy alternative, melted
- 1 teaspoon vanilla extract

FOR THE TOPPING

- 50 grams cane sugar or granulated sugar
- 100 grams light brown sugar
- 1 tablespoon Dutch-process cocoa powder
- ¼ teaspoon salt
- 1 cup boiling water

Directions:

TO MAKE THE COBBLER

Step 1

Preheat the oven to 350°F. Grease a 9-by-9-inch baking pan with shortening.

Step 2

In a medium bowl, whisk the flour, arrowroot, baking powder, cocoa powder, salt, xanthan gum, and sugar to combine. Using a spatula, stir in the milk, melted butter, and vanilla, mixing just until combined.

Step 3

Spread the mixture into the prepared pan.

TO MAKE THE TOPPING

Step 4

In a small bowl, whisk the cane sugar, brown sugar, cocoa powder, and salt to combine. Sprinkle the topping over the batter. Do not stir.

Step 5

Pour the boiling water evenly on top of the batter and topping. Do not stir.

Step 6

Bake for 30 minutes, or until the top is almost set. The cake should rise to the top and a creamy layer will form at the bottom. Serve warm.

Step 7

Keep leftovers covered and refrigerated for up to 3 days. Reheat to serve.

Pear Pecan Crisp

MAKES 1 (9-BY-9-INCH) CRISP

Prep time: 15 minutes

Cook time: 25 minutes

Ingredients:

- Shortening, for preparing the pan

FOR THE FILLING

- 32 grams All-Purpose Flour Blend
- 2 tablespoons light brown sugar
- 1 teaspoon vanilla extract
- 1 teaspoon ground cinnamon
- ¼ teaspoon xanthan gum
- ¼ teaspoon salt
- 6 firm-ripe pears, peeled and cut into thin, bite-size pieces
- 1 tablespoon fresh lemon juice

FOR THE TOPPING

- 32 grams All-Purpose Flour Blend
- 100 grams light brown sugar
- 50 grams certified gluten-free rolled oats
- 32 grams chopped pecans
- ¼ teaspoon xanthan gum
- 5 tablespoons plus 1 teaspoon butter or nondairy alternative, melted

Directions:

Step 1

Preheat the oven to 375°F. Grease a 9-by-9-inch pan with shortening.

TO MAKE THE FILLING

Step 2

In a small bowl, whisk the flour, brown sugar, vanilla, cinnamon, xanthan gum, and salt to combine.

Step 3

In a medium bowl, combine the pears and lemon juice. Add the flour mixture and, using a spatula, gently fold until the pear pieces are coated.

Step 4

Spread the filling in the prepared pan.

TO MAKE THE TOPPING

Step 5

In a medium bowl, whisk the flour, brown sugar, oats, pecans, and xanthan gum to combine. Using a spoon or spatula, stir in the melted butter. Evenly sprinkle the topping over the pears.

Step 6

Bake for 20 to 25 minutes, until the pears are tender and the crust is golden.

Step 7

Serve warm. Refrigerate leftovers, covered, for up to 3 days. Reheat to serve.

Classic Cheesecake

MAKES 1 (9-INCH) CHEESECAKE

Prep time: 1 hour

Cook time: about 3 hours, plus overnight chilling

Ingredients:

FOR THE CRUST

- 95 grams All-Purpose Flour Blend, plus more for dusting
- ¼ teaspoon xanthan gum
- ¼ teaspoon salt
- 8 tablespoons (1 stick) butter or nondairy alternative
- 50 grams cane sugar or granulated sugar
- 1 large egg yolk
- 1 teaspoon vanilla extract

FOR THE CHEESECAKE FILLING

- 4 (8-ounce) packages cream cheese or nondairy alternative, room temperature
- 300 grams cane sugar or granulated sugar
- 80 grams vanilla Greek yogurt or nondairy alternative
- 1 tablespoon vanilla extract
- 2 large egg yolks
- 4 large eggs

Directions:

TO MAKE THE CRUST

Step 1

Line the bottom of a 9-inch springform pan with aluminum foil and dust with a bit of flour. The foil should wrap around the entire bottom portion of the pan, including the outside.

Step 2

In a small bowl, whisk the flour, xanthan gum, and salt to combine.

Step 3

In a large bowl, using a whisk or handheld electric mixer, mix the butter, sugar, egg yolk, and vanilla until combined. Add the flour mixture and mix until a sticky dough forms.

Step 4

Transfer the dough to the prepared pan and dust a bit more flour on top so it doesn't stick to your fingers. Flatten the dough into a 6-inch-diameter disk, cover with plastic wrap, and chill for 30 minutes.

Step 5

Position an oven rack in the third lowest position and preheat the oven to 350°F.

Step 6

Release the clamp from the pan and remove the sides. Place a small piece of parchment paper over the chilled dough and use a rolling pin to stretch the dough to reach the edges of the pan. Work the edges so the dough fits well. Replace the sides of the pan, and tighten the clamp. Use your fingertips to push the dough up the sides just a little.

Step 7

Bake for 10 minutes. Remove from the oven but leave the oven on. Leave the oven rack where it is, but increase the oven temperature to 500°F.

Step 8

Let the crust cool for at least 10 minutes before preparing the cheesecake filling.

TO MAKE THE CHEESECAKE FILLING

Step 9

In a large bowl, using a whisk or handheld electric mixer, beat the cream cheese until smooth and creamy. Add the sugar, yogurt, and vanilla and mix again to combine. Add the egg yolks only and mix again.

Step 10

Add the whole eggs, 2 at a time, mixing after each set and stopping to scrape down the bowl as needed, also giving the bottom of the bowl a stir to make sure all the cream cheese is incorporated. Pour the batter over the cooled crust.

Step 11

Bake for 10 minutes, then (without opening the oven) reduce the oven temperature to 200°F and bake for 2 hours 30 minutes. The edges will be golden but the center may not be quite set. If you have an instant-read thermometer, the internal temperature should read 165°F.

Step 12

Let the cake sit in the pan at room temperature for 2 hours. Cover it with plastic wrap and refrigerate overnight.

Step 13

To remove the cake from the pan, run a butter knife along the outside of the cake to detach it from the sides. Release the clamp and remove the sides. Refrigerate, covered, for up to 4 days.

Triple-Layer Birthday Cake with Buttercream Frosting

MAKES 1 (9-INCH) THREE-LAYER FROSTED CAKE

Prep time: 30 minutes
Cook time: 30 minutes

Ingredients:

FOR THE CAKE

- Shortening, for preparing the pans
- 375 grams All-Purpose Flour Blend, plus more for dusting
- 62 grams arrowroot
- 1 tablespoon baking powder
- 1½ teaspoons xanthan gum
- 1 teaspoon baking soda
- ½ teaspoon salt
- 3 large eggs
- 2 large egg whites
- 400 grams cane sugar or granulated sugar
- 1½ cups whole milk or coconut milk beverage
- 1 cup avocado oil or canola oil
- 1 tablespoon vanilla extract
- 1 teaspoon apple cider vinegar

FOR THE BUTTERCREAM FROSTING
- 205 grams shortening
- 8 tablespoons (1 stick) butter or nondairy alternative
- 720 grams powdered sugar
- 2 teaspoons vanilla extract
- ¼ cup heavy cream or coconut cream

Directions:

TO MAKE THE CAKE

Step 1

Preheat the oven to 350°F. Grease three 9-inch springform pans with shortening. Sprinkle a little flour inside and tap the pans to spread the flour evenly around each pan.

Step 2

In a medium bowl, whisk the flour, arrowroot, baking powder, xanthan gum, baking soda, and salt to combine.

Step 3

In a small bowl, whisk the whole eggs to combine.

Step 4

In a large bowl, using a handheld electric mixer, whip the egg whites until soft peak forms. Add the cane sugar and beaten eggs to the egg whites and mix for 1 minute.

Step 5

Add the milk, oil, vanilla, and vinegar. Mix well. With the mixer on low speed, mix in the flour in 3 additions, stopping to scrape down the bowl, as needed.

Step 6

Evenly divide the batter between the prepared pans.

Step 7

Bake for 25 to 30 minutes, or until a toothpick inserted into the center of a cake comes out clean.

Step 8

Let the cakes cool in the pans for at least 15 minutes. Release the clamp from each pan and remove the sides. Transfer the cakes and plates to a wire rack to cool completely.

Step 9

Using a large serrated knife, cut off the thin domed layer from the top of each cake. Creating a flat surface will help the cakes stack well.

TO MAKE THE BUTTERCREAM FROSTING

Step 10

In a large bowl, using a handheld electric mixer on medium speed, cream together the shortening and butter. Add the powdered sugar and vanilla. Mix, while slowly adding the heavy cream, until smooth and creamy.

Step 11

Frost the cake layers and outside of the cake as desired. Refrigerate leftovers, covered, for up to 5 days.

Chocolate Crack Pie

MAKES 1 (9-INCH) PIE

Prep time: 30 minutes, plus 30 minutes to chill
Cook time: 40 minutes

Ingredients:
- Shortening, for preparing the pan
- 1 single Perfect Piecrust
- 125 grams All-Purpose Flour Blend
- 100 grams cane sugar or granulated sugar
- 100 grams light brown sugar
- ½ teaspoon xanthan gum
- 12 tablespoons (1½ sticks) butter or nondairy alternative
- 90 grams semisweet chocolate chips or nondairy alternative
- 2 large eggs
- 2 tablespoons whole milk or coconut milk beverage

Directions:

Step 1

Grease a 9-inch pie plate with shortening.

Step 2

Fit the piecrust into the prepared pie plate. Shape the edges. Refrigerate for at least 30 minutes.

Step 3

In a small bowl, whisk the flour, cane sugar, brown sugar, and xanthan gum to combine.

Step 4

Preheat the oven to 350°F.

Step 5

In a small saucepan, melt the butter over low heat. Add the chocolate chips. Cook, stirring, until melted. Remove the pan from the heat. Using a wooden spoon, immediately stir in the flour mixture until combined. Let stand 3 minutes to cool.

Step 6

Stir in the eggs and milk until smooth and creamy. Pour the filling into the chilled piecrust. If the oven is still preheating, place a piece of parchment paper on top of the pie and refrigerate it until the oven is ready.

Step 7

Bake for 35 to 40 minutes. or until the center does not jiggle.

Step 8

Let the pie cool completely before serving. Keep leftovers covered at room temperature, or refrigerate, for up to 5 days.

Perfect Piecrust

MAKES 1 (9-INCH) DOUBLE PIECRUST OR 2 (9-INCH) SINGLE PIECRUSTS

Prep time: 1 hour

Ingredients:

- 136 grams chilled shortening
- 8 tablespoons (1 stick) butter or nondairy alternative
- 250 grams <u>All-Purpose Flour Blend</u>, plus more for dusting
- 63 grams brown rice flour
- 63 grams sorghum flour
- 1½ teaspoons xanthan gum

- 1 teaspoon salt
- 1 large egg
- 1 tablespoon apple cider vinegar
- 2 to 3 tablespoons ice-cold water

Directions:

Step 1

Freeze the shortening and butter for at least 30 minutes.

Step 2

Place two sheets of parchment paper on a work surface and dust them with the all-purpose flour.

Step 3

In a medium bowl, whisk the all-purpose flour, rice flour, sorghum flour, xanthan gum, and salt to combine.

Step 4

Cut the cold butter into pieces and add it and the cold shortening to the flour mixture. Using a pastry cutter, cut the fats into the flour until a crumbly mixture forms. Add the egg, vinegar, and 2 tablespoons of ice-cold water. Mix the dough, adding the remaining 1 tablespoon of ice-cold water, as needed, until a smooth dough forms.

Step 5

Divide the dough into 2 portions. Place one portion on a floured sheet of parchment and put the second sheet of parchment on top. Roll the dough into a 12-inch round a little less than ¼ inch thick.

Step 6

Remove the top sheet of parchment and flip the dough into the pie plate. Push down from the edges (not the middle) to create slack. Gently fit the dough into the bottom and sides of the plate. Remove the remaining piece of parchment. Smooth and crimp the edges of the crust, as desired. Refrigerate for at least 30 minutes before baking.

Step 7

Repeat steps 5 and 6 with the second dough portion either to make a second bottom crust or to roll it into an 11-inch round for a top crust.

Blueberry Crumble Slab Pie

MAKES 1 (9-BY-13-INCH) SLAB PIE

Prep time: 50 minutes
Cook time: 30 minutes

Ingredients:

FOR THE CRUST

- Shortening, for preparing the pan
- 313 grams All-Purpose Flour Blend , plus more for dusting
- 1 teaspoon xanthan gum
- 1 teaspoon salt
- 12 tablespoons (1½ sticks) cold butter or nondairy alternative
- 8 to 10 tablespoons ice-cold water

FOR THE FILLING

- 200 grams cane sugar or granulated sugar
- 32 grams All-Purpose Flour Blend

- ¼ teaspoon xanthan gum
- 600 grams blueberries
- 1 tablespoon fresh lemon juice

FOR THE CRUMBLE TOPPING
- 100 grams certified gluten-free rolled oats
- 200 grams light brown sugar
- 62 grams All-Purpose Flour Blend
- 1 teaspoon ground cinnamon
- ¼ teaspoon xanthan gum
- 8 tablespoons (1 stick) butter or nondairy alternative
- 62 grams chopped pecans (optional)

Directions:

TO MAKE THE CRUST

Step 1

Line a 9-by-13-inch jelly-roll pan with aluminum foil and lightly grease it with shortening. Place two sheets of parchment paper on a work surface and dust them with flour.

Step 2

In a medium bowl, whisk the flour, xanthan gum, and salt to combine.

Step 3

Cut the butter into small pieces and add it to the flour mixture. Using a pastry cutter, cut the butter into the flour mixture until crumbs form.

Step 4

Add 2 tablespoons of ice-cold water as you form the dough by hand. Continue to add the water, 1 tablespoon at a time, until the dough is smooth. Transfer the dough to the floured work surface and divide it into 2 portions.

Step 5

Roll 1 portion of the dough between the two parchment sheets to about ⅛ inch thick. Remove the top sheet of parchment. Flip the dough into one side of the prepared pan using the technique from my Perfect Piecrust (step 6).

Step 6

Repeat rolling the second dough portion and flip it into the other side of the pan so both pieces overlap in the center. Use your fingers to connect them and smooth the surface. Trim and crimp the edges. Refrigerate the crust for at least 30 minutes while you prepare the filling and topping.

TO MAKE THE FILLING

Step 7

In a small bowl, whisk the sugar, flour, and xanthan gum to combine.

Step 8

Place the blueberries in a large bowl and sprinkle them with lemon juice. Stir to be sure all the berries are coated in the juice. Add the flour mixture and stir again to coat.

TO MAKE THE CRUMBLE TOPPING

Step 9

Preheat the oven to 375°F.

Step 10

In a medium bowl, whisk the oats, brown sugar, flour, cinnamon, and xanthan gum to combine. Using a pastry cutter, cut the butter into the flour mixture until crumbs form. Stir in the pecans (if using).

Step 11

Remove the chilled crust from the refrigerator and pour the filling over it. Sprinkle the crumble on top.

Step 12

Bake for 30 minutes, or until the blueberries are bubbling.

Step 13

Serve warm or cold. Keep leftovers covered at room temperature for 2 days, or refrigerate for up to 4 days.

Cinnamon Roll Pancakes

MAKES 6 PANCAKES

Prep time: 15 minutes

Cook time: 20 minutes

Ingredients:

FOR THE CINNAMON SWIRL

- 5 tablespoons light brown sugar
- 3 tablespoons butter or nondairy alternative, melted
- 2 teaspoons ground cinnamon

FOR THE PANCAKES

- Gluten-free cooking spray
- 125 grams All-Purpose Flour Blend
- 2 tablespoons cane sugar or granulated sugar
- 1½ teaspoons baking powder
- ½ teaspoon salt
- ¼ teaspoon xanthan gum
- ¼ teaspoon baking soda
- ¼ teaspoon ground cinnamon
- ¾ cup whole milk or coconut milk beverage
- 1 large egg
- 2 tablespoons avocado oil or canola oil
- 1 teaspoon vanilla extract

FOR THE GLAZE

- 200 grams powdered sugar
- 2 tablespoons whole milk or coconut milk beverage
- ½ teaspoon vanilla extract

Directions:

TO MAKE THE CINNAMON SWIRL

Step 1

In a small bowl, stir together the brown sugar, melted butter, and cinnamon until blended.

TO MAKE THE PANCAKES

Step 2

Heat a skillet or griddle over medium heat and coat it with cooking spray. (Because these pancakes have the delicate cinnamon swirl, I do not recommend using butter to coat the pan.)

Step 3

In a medium bowl, whisk the flour, sugar, baking powder, salt, xanthan gum, baking soda, and cinnamon to combine. Add the milk, egg, oil, and vanilla and stir to combine. Let the batter sit for 5 minutes.

Step 4

Add the cinnamon swirl to a piping bag or plastic bag. Snip the tip about ¼ inch wide and place the bag in a large glass with the tip bent up so the swirl doesn't spill out.

Step 5

Place ¼ cup of batter for each pancake in the hot skillet. Do not overcrowd the skillet. Pipe a swirl of the cinnamon mixture onto each pancake. Cook for 3 minutes, or until bubbles form and pop. Carefully flip the pancake and cook for 2 to 3 minutes more, or until set, watching closely to avoid burning the cinnamon swirl.

Step 6

Repeat with the remaining batter and cinnamon swirl, wiping the skillet clean between batches if the swirl makes it too sticky, and adding more cooking spray as needed.

TO MAKE THE GLAZE

Step 7

In a small bowl, whisk the powdered sugar, milk, and vanilla until smooth.

Step 8

Drizzle the glaze over each pancake and serve. These are best served warm the same day.

The Infamous Pumpkin Muffins

MAKES 12 MUFFINS
Prep time: 10 minutes
Cook time: 25 minutes

Ingredients:

- 250 grams All-Purpose Flour Blend
- 2 teaspoons baking powder
- 1½ teaspoons ground cinnamon
- 1 teaspoon pumpkin pie spice
- 1 teaspoon xanthan gum
- ½ teaspoon baking soda
- ½ teaspoon salt
- 100 grams light brown sugar
- 2 large eggs
- ½ cup avocado oil or canola oil
- ½ cup maple syrup
- 2 teaspoons vanilla extract
- 225 grams pumpkin puree
- Cane sugar or granulated sugar, for sprinkling (optional)

Directions:

Step 1

Preheat the oven to 425°F. Line a 12-cup muffin tin with cupcake liners.

Step 2

In a medium bowl, whisk the flour, baking powder, cinnamon, pumpkin pie spice, xanthan gum, baking soda, and salt to combine.

Step 3

In another medium bowl, whisk the brown sugar, eggs, oil, maple syrup, and vanilla until smooth.

Step 4

Add the flour mixture to the egg mixture and mix with a rubber spatula until combined. Fold in the pumpkin. Do not overmix. Evenly divide the batter between the prepared muffin cups. Sprinkle the top of each muffin with sugar (if using).

Step 5

Bake for 5 minutes to let the muffins set, then (without opening the oven) reduce the oven temperature to 350°F and bake for 20 minutes more, or until a toothpick inserted into the center of a muffin comes out clean.

Step 6

Let the muffins cool in the pan for 15 minutes, then transfer them to a wire rack. Serve warm or let cool completely. Store leftovers in an airtight container at room temperature for up to 3 days.

Double-Chocolate Chunk Muffins

MAKES 12 MUFFINS
Prep time: 15 minutes
Cook time: 25 minutes

Ingredients:

- 250 grams All-Purpose Flour Blend
- 75 grams Dutch-process cocoa powder
- 2 teaspoons baking powder
- 1 teaspoon xanthan gum
- ½ teaspoon baking soda
- ½ teaspoon salt
- 200 grams cane sugar or granulated sugar
- 100 grams light brown sugar
- 2 large eggs
- 240 grams vanilla Greek yogurt or nondairy alternative
- ½ cup avocado oil or canola oil
- 2 teaspoons vanilla extract
- 270 grams semisweet chocolate chunks or nondairy alternative

Directions:

Step 1

Preheat the oven to 425°F. Line a 12-cup muffin tin with cupcake liners.

Step 2

In a medium bowl, whisk the flour, cocoa powder, baking powder, xanthan gum, baking soda, and salt to combine.

Step 3

In another medium bowl, using a whisk or handheld electric mixer, mix the cane sugar, brown sugar, eggs, yogurt, oil, and vanilla until well combined.

Step 4

Add half the flour mixture to the yogurt mixture, mix on low speed, then add the remaining half of the flour mixture, mixing just until a batter is formed. Do not overmix.

Step 5

Using a spatula, fold in the chocolate chunks. Evenly divide the batter between the prepared muffin cups.

Step 6

Bake for 5 minutes to let the muffins set, then (without opening the oven) reduce the oven temperature to 350°F and bake for 20 minutes more, or until a toothpick inserted into the center of a muffin comes out clean.

Step 7

Let the muffins cool in the pan for 10 minutes, then transfer them to a wire rack to cool completely.

Step 8

Keep the muffins covered for about 3 days at room temperature, or refrigerate for up to 5 days.

Sweet Blackberry Muffins

MAKES 12 MUFFINS
Prep time: 15 minutes
Cook time: 25 minutes

Ingredients:

- 250 grams All-Purpose Flour Blend , plus 2 tablespoons, divided
- 2 teaspoons baking powder
- 1 teaspoon xanthan gum
- 1 teaspoon ground cinnamon
- ½ teaspoon ground nutmeg
- ½ teaspoon baking soda
- ½ teaspoon salt
- 100 grams cane sugar or granulated sugar, plus 4 teaspoons, divided
- 100 grams light brown sugar
- 6 tablespoons butter or nondairy alternative
- ½ cup whole milk or coconut milk beverage
- 80 grams vanilla Greek yogurt or nondairy alternative
- 2 large eggs
- 2 teaspoons vanilla extract
- ¼ teaspoon orange extract
- 230 grams blackberries

Directions:

Step 1

Preheat the oven to 425°F. Line a 12-cup muffin tin with cupcake liners.

Step 2

In a medium bowl, whisk 250 grams of flour, the baking powder, xanthan gum, cinnamon, nutmeg, baking soda, and salt to combine.

Step 3

In a small bowl, using a handheld electric mixer on medium speed, cream together 100 grams of cane sugar, the brown sugar, and butter until smooth. Beat in the milk, yogurt, eggs, vanilla, and orange extract until combined.

Step 4

In another small bowl, toss the blackberries with the remaining 2 tablespoons of flour and 1 teaspoon of cane sugar until well coated.

Step 5

Using a spatula, add the flour mixture to the butter mixture and mix until combined. Do not overmix. Gently fold in the blackberries. Evenly divide the batter between the prepared muffin cups. Smooth the tops of each muffin with your finger and sprinkle the remaining 3 teaspoons of sugar over the muffins.

Step 6

Bake for 5 minutes to let the muffins set, then (without opening the oven) reduce the oven temperature to 350°F and bake for 20 minutes more, or until a toothpick inserted into the center of a muffin comes out clean.

Step 7

Let the muffins cool in the pan for 10 minutes, then transfer them to a wire rack to cool completely. Keep the muffins covered for about 3 days at room temperature, or refrigerate, covered, for up to 5 days.

Oatmeal Blueberry Muffins

MAKES 12 MUFFINS
Prep time: 40 minutes
Cook time: 25 minutes

Ingredients:

- 100 grams certified gluten-free rolled oats
- 1 cup whole milk or coconut milk beverage
- 1 teaspoon ground cinnamon
- 250 grams All-Purpose Flour Blend
- 2 teaspoons baking powder
- 1 teaspoon xanthan gum
- ½ teaspoon baking soda
- ½ teaspoon salt
- ½ cup avocado oil or canola oil
- ½ cup maple syrup
- 2 large eggs
- 2 teaspoons vanilla extract
- 100 grams blueberries

Directions:

Step 1

In a small bowl, stir together the oats, milk, and cinnamon. Let sit for 20 minutes, or until most of the milk has been absorbed. If needed, stir the oats and let soak for 10 minutes more.

Step 2

Preheat the oven to 425°F. Line a 12-cup muffin tin with cupcake liners.

Step 3

In a medium bowl, whisk the flour, baking powder, xanthan gum, baking soda, and salt to combine.

Step 4

In another medium bowl, whisk the oil, maple syrup, eggs, and vanilla until combined. Using a spatula, mix in the flour mixture. Add the soaked oats and mix again to combine. Gently fold in the blueberries. Evenly divide the batter between the prepared muffin cups.

Step 5

Bake for 5 minutes to let the muffins set, then (without opening the oven) reduce the oven temperature to 350°F and bake 20 minutes more, or until a toothpick inserted into the center of a muffin comes out clean.

Step 6

Let the muffins cool in the pan for 10 minutes, then transfer them to a wire rack to cool completely. Keep the muffins covered for about 3 days at room temperature or refrigerate for up to 5 days.

Thin Mint Cupcakes

MAKES 12 CUPCAKES

Prep time: 1 hour
Cook time: about 20 minutes

Ingredients:

FOR THE CUPCAKES

- 95 grams All-Purpose Flour Blend
- 50 grams Dutch-process cocoa powder
- 1 tablespoon arrowroot
- ¾ teaspoon baking powder
- ½ teaspoon baking soda
- ½ teaspoon xanthan gum
- ¼ teaspoon salt
- 150 grams cane sugar or granulated sugar
- 50 grams light brown sugar
- 2 large eggs
- ⅓ cup avocado oil or canola oil
- ½ cup whole milk or coconut milk beverage
- 2 teaspoons vanilla extract
- ½ teaspoon apple cider vinegar
- ½ recipe Thin Mint Copycat Cookies, prepared through step 4 and rolled into 12 balls

FOR THE MINT FROSTING

- 136 grams shortening
- ¼ teaspoon peppermint extract
- 2 drops green food coloring
- 480 grams powdered sugar
- 4 tablespoons whole milk or coconut milk beverage

Directions:

TO MAKE THE CUPCAKES

Step 1

Preheat the oven to 350°F. Line a 12-cup muffin tin with cupcake liners.

Step 2

In a medium bowl, whisk the flour, cocoa powder, arrowroot, baking powder, baking soda, xanthan gum, and salt to combine.

Step 3
In a large bowl, using a whisk or handheld electric mixer, mix the cane sugar, brown sugar, eggs, oil, milk, vanilla, and vinegar. Beat in the flour mixture in two additions, mixing on low speed to blend and stopping to scrape down the bowl as needed, and making sure there are no brown sugar clumps. The batter should be thick.

Step 4
Place 1 cookie dough ball into each prepared muffin cup. Evenly divide the batter over each, filling each cup no more than two-thirds full.

Step 5
Bake for 18 to 20 minutes, or until a toothpick inserted in the side of a cupcake comes out clean. (Be careful to avoid the cookie dough center when testing for doneness.)

Step 6
Let the cupcakes cool in the pan for at least 10 minutes, then transfer to a wire rack to cool completely.

TO MAKE THE MINT FROSTING

Step 7
In a large bowl, using a handheld electric mixer on medium speed, cream the shortening.

Step 8
Add the mint extract, food coloring, and powdered sugar and mix to combine. While mixing, add the milk by the tablespoon and mix until smooth and creamy.

Step 9
Frost the cupcakes. Keep leftovers in an airtight container at room temperature for up to 4 days.

Very Strawberry Cupcakes

MAKES 12 CUPCAKES

Prep time: 1 hour 45 minutes
Cook time: 42 minutes

Ingredients:

FOR THE STRAWBERRY FILLING
- 250 grams sliced fresh strawberries
- 2 tablespoons cane sugar or granulated sugar

FOR THE CUPCAKES
- 207 grams All-Purpose Flour Blend
- 2 tablespoons arrowroot
- 1 teaspoon xanthan gum
- 1 teaspoon baking soda
- ¼ teaspoon salt
- 8 tablespoons (1 stick) butter or nondairy alternative
- 200 grams cane sugar or granulated sugar
- 3 large egg whites
- 60 grams vanilla Greek yogurt or nondairy alternative
- 2 teaspoons vanilla extract
- ⅓ cup whole milk or coconut milk beverage

FOR THE STRAWBERRY FROSTING

- 34 grams freeze-dried strawberries
- 240 grams powdered sugar
- 68 grams shortening
- 2 to 3 tablespoons whole milk or coconut milk beverage
- 1 teaspoon vanilla extract

Directions:

TO MAKE THE STRAWBERRY FILLING

Step 1

In a small saucepan, combine the strawberries and sugar. Bring to a simmer over medium heat and cook for about 20 minutes, stirring occasionally to prevent burning. The strawberries will reduce and thicken. Transfer to a bowl, cover with plastic wrap, and refrigerate for at least 1 hour.

TO MAKE THE CUPCAKES

Step 2

Preheat the oven to 350°F. Line a 12-cup muffin tin with cupcake liners.

Step 3

In a small bowl, whisk the flour, arrowroot, xanthan gum, baking soda, and salt to combine.

Step 4

In a large bowl, using a handheld electric mixer on medium speed, cream together the butter and cane sugar. Add the egg whites and mix until combined, stopping to scrape down the bowl as needed. Add the yogurt, vanilla, and milk. Mix again.

Step 5

Using a spatula, scrape the sides and the bottom of the bowl to make sure all ingredients at the bottom are mixed in. With the mixer on low speed, slowly add the flour mixture. The batter will look curdled. That's okay.

Step 6

Using a spatula, fold in ½ cup of the strawberry filling (you may have a bit extra leftover) until it is evenly spread through the batter. Evenly divide the batter between the prepared muffin cups, filling each two-thirds full. Do not overfill.

Step 7

Bake for 20 to 22 minutes, or until a toothpick inserted into the center of a cupcake comes out clean.

Step 8

Let the cupcakes cool completely before frosting.

TO MAKE THE STRAWBERRY FROSTING

Step 9

In a food processor, pulse the freeze-dried strawberries to form a fine powder.

Step 10

In a large bowl, using a handheld electric mixer, beat together the powdered sugar, shortening, strawberry powder, milk, and vanilla until smooth.

Step 11

Transfer the frosting to a piping bag with your choice of tip. Frost the cupcakes. Refrigerate leftovers, covered, for up to 5 days.

Fudgy Chocolate Cupcakes

MAKES 12 CUPCAKES

Prep time: 30 minutes

Cook time: 30 minutes

Ingredients:

FOR THE CUPCAKES

- 190 grams All-Purpose Flour Blend
- 25 grams Dutch-process cocoa powder
- 1 teaspoon baking powder
- ½ teaspoon xanthan gum
- ¼ teaspoon salt
- 155 grams dark chocolate chips or nondairy alternative
- 6 tablespoons butter or nondairy alternative
- 200 grams cane sugar or granulated sugar
- 160 grams vanilla Greek yogurt or nondairy alternative
- 2 large eggs
- 2 teaspoons vanilla extract

FOR THE GANACHE

- 270 grams semisweet chocolate chips or nondairy alternative
- ¼ cup coconut oil, melted

Directions:

TO MAKE THE CUPCAKES

Step 1

Preheat the oven to 350°F. Line a 12-cup muffin tin with cupcake liners.

Step 2

In a medium bowl, whisk the flour, cocoa powder, baking powder, xanthan gum, and salt to combine.

Step 3

In a small saucepan, combine the chocolate chips and butter. Melt over low heat, stirring constantly until smooth. Set aside.

Step 4

In a large bowl, using a handheld electric mixer, beat the sugar, yogurt, eggs, and vanilla until well mixed. Add the chocolate mixture and continue beating. Beat in the flour mixture in two additions. Mix until combined. The batter will be very thick.

Step 5

Evenly divide the batter between the prepared muffin cups. With a slightly damp finger, smooth the top of each.

Step 6

Bake for 18 to 20 minutes, or until a toothpick inserted into a cupcake comes out clean.

Step 7

Let the cupcakes cool completely before frosting.

TO MAKE THE GANACHE

Step 8

In a small saucepan, combine the chocolate chips and coconut oil. Melt over low heat, stirring until smooth.

Step 9

Dip the top of each cupcake in the chocolate ganache. Once you have dipped all 12 cupcakes, dip them again. Set aside to let the chocolate ganache set and solidify.

Step 10

Keep leftovers covered at room temperature for up to 3 days.

Samoa Donuts

MAKES 12 DONUTS

Prep time: 30 minutes

Cook time: about 1 hour

Ingredients:

- 100 grams shredded coconut

FOR THE DONUTS

- Shortening, for preparing the pans
- 282 grams All-Purpose Flour Blend
- 150 grams cane sugar or granulated sugar
- 2 teaspoons baking powder
- 1 teaspoon salt
- ½ teaspoon xanthan gum
- ½ teaspoon ground cinnamon
- 1 cup buttermilk, or 1 cup coconut milk beverage plus 1 tablespoon apple cider vinegar (see here)
- ½ cup avocado oil or canola oil, plus more for frying
- 2 large eggs
- 2 teaspoons vanilla extract

FOR THE CHOCOLATE DRIZZLE

- 360 grams semisweet chocolate chips or nondairy alternative
- 1 tablespoon coconut oil

FOR THE CARAMEL SAUCE

- 100 grams cane sugar or granulated sugar
- 3 tablespoons butter or nondairy alternative
- ¼ cup heavy cream or coconut cream
- ½ teaspoon salt

Directions:

Step 1

Preheat the oven to 325°F. Line a baking sheet with parchment paper.

Step 2

Spread the coconut into a thin layer on the prepared baking sheet. Toast for 5 to 7 minutes, or until golden. Set the toasted coconut aside.

TO MAKE THE DONUTS

Step 3

Increase the oven temperature to 425°F. Grease two 6-well donut pans with shortening.

Step 4

In a large bowl, whisk the flour, sugar, baking powder, salt, xanthan gum, and cinnamon to combine.

Step 5

In another large bowl, using a handheld electric mixer, beat the buttermilk, oil, eggs, and vanilla. Add the flour mixture to the wet ingredients and beat until combined. The batter will be slightly runny.

Step 6

Transfer the batter to a piping bag or plastic bag. Cut the tip and evenly fill the prepared donut wells with batter.

Step 7

Bake for 9 minutes, then (without opening the oven) reduce the temperature to 350°F and bake for 5 to 7 minutes more, or until a toothpick inserted into the center of a donut comes out clean.

Step 8

Let the donuts cool in the pans for 10 minutes, then transfer to a wire rack to cool completely.

Step 9

In a skillet, heat ⅛ inch of oil over medium heat. You'll know the oil is ready when a drop of water sizzles in it. Place 2 or 3 donuts facedown (lighter-side down) in the oil and flash-fry for 2 to 3 minutes, or until the donuts sizzle and pick up a little color. Watch closely to prevent burning. Flip and flash-fry the other side for 1 to 2 minutes. Transfer the donuts back to the rack to cool.

Step 10

Repeat with the remaining donuts. As the oil gets hotter, the donuts will need less time. Be careful not to burn them. Add more oil, as needed.

TO MAKE THE CHOCOLATE DRIZZLE

Step 11

Line a baking sheet with parchment paper.

Step 12

In a small saucepan, melt the chocolate chips over low heat. Stir in the coconut oil until smooth.

Step 13

Dip the underside of each donut in the chocolate and transfer to the prepared baking sheet to set. Set aside any remaining chocolate.

TO MAKE THE CARAMEL SAUCE

Step 14

In a small saucepan, melt the sugar over medium heat, stirring constantly. If your sugar is not melting, increase the heat just a bit. Keep stirring so the sugar does not burn (this can happen quickly).

Step 15

Remove the pan from the heat and slowly add the butter, stirring constantly and being careful not to splatter hot sugar.

Step 16

Slowly stir in the cream. Return the pan to low heat. When everything is incorporated, increase the heat and bring to a boil. Boil for 1 to 2 minutes. Remove from the heat and stir in the salt. Let the sauce cool for about 5 minutes.

Step 17

In a large bowl, stir together a few tablespoons of caramel sauce and the toasted coconut.

Step 18

Spread a thin layer of caramel sauce on top of each donut (opposite the chocolate). The caramel will solidify quickly. Top each donut with an equal amount of the caramel coconut, pressing it down to stick.

Step 19

Drizzle the donuts with the remaining melted chocolate (you may need to reheat it). Allow the topping to set for about 30 minutes.

Delicious Donut Holes

MAKES 34 DONUT HOLES

Prep time: 1 hour 15 minutes
Cook time: 15 minutes

Ingredients:

- 375 grams All-Purpose Flour Blend
- 1 teaspoon xanthan gum
- 1 teaspoon salt
- ½ teaspoon ground cinnamon
- 1 cup warm (100° to 110°F) whole milk or coconut milk beverage
- 50 grams cane sugar or granulated sugar
- 1 (7-gram) packet instant (fast-acting) yeast
- 1 large egg
- 1 teaspoon apple cider vinegar
- Oil or shortening, for frying
- Double batch of glaze (from Cinnamon Roll Pancakes)

Directions:

Step 1

In a medium bowl, whisk the flour, xanthan gum, salt, and cinnamon to combine.

Step 2

In a large bowl, combine the warm milk, sugar, and yeast. Give it a stir and let sit for 5 minutes.

Step 3

Add the egg and vinegar and, using a handheld electric mixer, mix well. Add the flour mixture to the wet ingredients and mix to form a wet dough. Cover the bowl with plastic wrap and let the dough rest for at least 1 hour.

Step 4

Place a paper towel over a wire rack and place the rack on a baking sheet. Pour 3 inches of oil into a deep, large heavy-bottomed pan and heat to 350°F over medium heat.

Step 5

Coat the inside of a 1-inch ice cream scoop with a little oil. Carefully scoop dough balls into the hot oil. Fry for 1 to 2 minutes, turning, until golden brown. Using a slotted spoon, transfer to the paper towel to drain. Let the donut holes cool for 10 minutes.

Step 6

Place the glaze in a large bowl and add the donut holes. Stir to coat on all sides. Using a slotted spoon, transfer them back to the rack to set for 1 hour before serving. Keep leftovers in an airtight container at room temperature for up to 3 days. Humidity levels in your house may cause the glaze to melt a bit.

Italian Zeppoli (Sfingi)

MAKES 40 ZEPPOLI
Prep time: about 4 hours

Cook time: 30 minutes

Ingredients:

FOR THE TOPPING

- 200 grams cane sugar or granulated sugar
- 1½ teaspoons ground cinnamon

FOR THE ZEPPOLI

- 296 grams Yukon Gold potatoes, peeled
- 250 grams All-Purpose Flour Blend
- ½ teaspoon xanthan gum
- ¼ teaspoon salt
- Grated zest of 1 lemon
- 1 (7-gram) packet instant (fast-acting) yeast
- 1 cup warm (100° to 110°F) water
- Oil or shortening, for frying

Directions:

TO MAKE THE TOPPING

Step 1

In a medium bowl, stir together the sugar and cinnamon. Set aside.

TO MAKE THE ZEPPOLI

Step 2

Bring a medium pot of water to a boil over high heat. Add the potatoes and boil for about 20 minutes, or until fork-tender. Drain, return to the pot, and, using a potato masher, mash them while hot. Let the potatoes cool.

Step 3

In a large bowl, whisk the flour, xanthan gum, salt, and lemon zest to combine.

Step 4

Using a ricer, rice the mashed potatoes into the flour mixture. Using your hands, toss everything together.

Step 5

In a small bowl, combine the yeast and warm water. Let sit for 5 minutes.

Step 6

Add the yeast mixture to the flour/potato mixture and, using your hands, form a very wet dough. Work the dough well for about 5 minutes, turning it multiple times. Cover the bowl with plastic wrap and let the dough rest for at least 3 hours.

Step 7

Pour 3 inches of oil into a large, deep heavy-bottomed pan and heat to 350°F over medium heat.

Step 8

Using a 1-inch ice cream scoop, carefully scoop dough balls into the hot oil. Cook for 3 to 4 minutes, or until puffed and golden. Using a slotted spoon, transfer them directly to the cinnamon sugar and toss to coat. Sfingi are best served warm the same day.

Cannoli

MAKES 12 CANNOLI

Prep time: 4 hours 30 minutes

Cook time: 20 minutes

Ingredients:

FOR THE SHELLS

- Shortening, for preparing the cannoli tubes
- 313 grams <u>All-Purpose Flour Blend</u> , plus more for dusting
- 1½ tablespoons cane sugar or granulated sugar
- 1 teaspoon xanthan gum
- ¼ teaspoon salt
- 2 tablespoons butter or nondairy alternative
- 2 large egg yolks
- ⅔ cup plus 1 tablespoon white wine or marsala
- Oil or shortening, for frying

FOR THE FILLING

- 1,500 grams ricotta
- 2 teaspoons vanilla extract
- 150 grams powdered sugar, plus more as needed

Directions:

TO START THE SHELLS

Step 1

Line a baking sheet with a silicone baking mat (so the shells don't roll around). Place two sheets of parchment paper on a work surface and dust them with flour. Grease 12 cannoli forms with shortening.

Step 2

In a medium bowl, whisk the flour, sugar, xanthan gum, and salt to combine.

Step 3

Cut the butter into small pieces and add it to the flour mixture along with the egg yolks. Using a pastry cutter, or handheld electric mixer, mix the dough until crumbly.

Step 4

Slowly add the wine, mixing until smooth. Transfer the dough to the floured work surface. Shape it into a 12-inch log. Cut the log into 6 (2-inch) pieces. Roll each portion between the two sheets of parchment to ⅛ inch thick.

Step 5

Using a 3-inch round cookie or biscuit cutter, cut out 1 round from each portion. Reroll the scraps and repeat. You should end up with 12 rounds (see Tip).

Step 6

Do one final pass with your rolling pin over all the dough rounds to thin them a bit. The rounds may look more like ovals. That's a good thing.

Step 7

Carefully wrap each dough round around a cannoli form (or a tube made from aluminum foil). Dip your fingertip in a little water to seal the seams. Do not wrap the dough too tightly or they will be difficult to remove after frying.

Step 8

Place all the cannoli shells on the prepared baking sheet and refrigerate for at least 4 hours.

Step 9

Line a colander with paper towels, place it over a large bowl, and spoon the ricotta into the lined colander. Set over a bowl and refrigerate to drain for about 1 hour.

TO MAKE THE FILLING

Step 10

In a large bowl, using a handheld electric mixer, beat the drained ricotta and vanilla for about 2 minutes until smooth and fluffy. Add the powdered sugar and mix until smooth and thick, adding more sugar if needed to thicken.

Step 11

Transfer the filling to a piping bag with tip of choice and keep refrigerated until the dough is done chilling.

TO FINISH THE CANNOLI

Step 12

Place a paper towel on top of a wire rack and place the rack on a baking sheet.

Step 13

In a large, deep heavy-bottomed pan, heat 3 inches of shortening to 350°F over medium heat.

Step 14

Working in batches, add the cannoli shells to the hot oil. Cook for 3 to 5 minutes, using tongs to gently move and roll them around, until golden brown. Transfer to the paper towel. Repeat with the remaining shells.

Step 15

Let the shells cool for 10 minutes before removing the cannoli forms.

Step 16

Fill the cannoli shells from both sides, making sure the middle gets filled. Dust the filled cannoli with powdered sugar. Refrigerate leftovers, covered, for up to 3 days.

Pepperoni Pizza Rolls

MAKES 12 PIZZA ROLLS

Prep time: 1 hour 15 minutes
Cook time: 30 minutes

Ingredients:

FOR THE CRUST

- 437 grams All-Purpose Flour Blend , plus more for dusting
- 2 teaspoons xanthan gum
- 1 teaspoon salt
- 1 tablespoon cane sugar or granulated sugar
- 1 (7-gram) packet instant (fast-acting) yeast
- 1⅓ cups (100° to 110°F) warm water
- 2 tablespoons olive oil
- ½ teaspoon apple cider vinegar

FOR THE FILLING

- ½ cup gluten-free pizza sauce
- 100 grams shredded mozzarella cheese or nondairy alternative, plus more for topping (optional)
- 1 (4-ounce) package sliced gluten-free pepperoni (I like Applegate brand), plus more diced for topping (optional)

Directions:
TO MAKE THE CRUST
Step 1

Position an oven rack in the lower third of the oven. Place two sheets of parchment paper on a work surface and dust them with flour.

Step 2

In a medium bowl, whisk the flour, xanthan gum, and salt to combine.

Step 3

In a large bowl, combine the sugar, yeast, and warm water. Give it a stir and let the mixture sit for 5 minutes.

Step 4

Add the oil and vinegar and give it another quick stir. Beat in the flour mixture in two additions and stir until a dough forms.

Step 5

Transfer the dough to the flour-dusted parchment and flatten it by hand. Place the second sheet of parchment on top and roll the dough to ⅛ to ¼ inch thick—the thinner, the better.

TO MAKE THE FILLING
Step 6

Line a baking sheet with parchment paper.

Step 7

Spread the pizza sauce evenly over the dough, leaving a ½-inch border. Cover with the cheese and arrange the pepperoni on top. Gently lift the edge closest to you and roll the pizza into a long log. Give it a gentle roll to seal the seam. Using a sharp knife, cut the roll into 12 pieces and place them on the prepared baking sheet. Cover loosely with plastic wrap and let them rest and rise for at least 1 hour.

Step 8

Preheat the oven to 475°F.

Step 9

Top the pizza rolls with more cheese (if using) and diced pepperoni (if using).

Step 10

Bake for 25 to 30 minutes, or until crisp.

Step 11

Let the rolls cool for about 5 minutes, then serve immediately. They are best served the same day. Refrigerate leftovers, covered, for up to 3 days. Reheat to serve.

Stromboli Pockets

MAKES 6 TO 8

Prep time: 1 hour 15 minutes
Cook time: 20 minutes

Ingredients:
FOR THE CRUST

- 375 grams All-Purpose Flour Blend , plus more for dusting
- 1 large egg
- 3 tablespoons olive oil, divided

- 2 teaspoons xanthan gum
- 1½ teaspoons salt
- 1 tablespoon cane sugar or granulated sugar
- 1 (7-gram) packet instant (fast-acting) yeast
- 1 cup warm (100° to 110°F) water
- 1 tablespoon honey
- ½ teaspoon apple cider vinegar

FOR THE POCKETS
- ¾ cup gluten-free pizza sauce
- 8 slices gluten-free salami
- 4 slices gluten-free deli ham
- 16 slices gluten-free pepperoni
- 100 grams shredded mozzarella cheese or nondairy alternative

Directions:

TO MAKE THE CRUST

Step 1
Position an oven rack in the lower third of the oven. Place two sheets of parchment paper on a work surface and dust them with flour. Line a baking sheet with parchment.

Step 2
In a small bowl, whisk the egg and 1 tablespoon water to create an egg wash. Pour 1 tablespoon of oil in another small bowl. Place the bowls next to the work surface.

Step 3
In a medium bowl, whisk the flour, xanthan gum, and salt to combine.

Step 4
In a large bowl, combine the sugar, yeast, and warm water. Give it a stir and let sit for 5 minutes.

Step 5
Add the remaining 2 tablespoons of oil, the honey, and vinegar and give it another quick stir. Stir in the flour mixture in two additions and stir until a dough forms.

Step 6
Transfer the dough to the floured work surface. Dip your fingertips in the oil bath and flatten the dough by hand. Divide it into 2 equal portions. Place the second sheet of parchment on top of one portion and roll the dough to ⅛ inch thick. You want this to be thin so the filling is prominent. Using a pizza cutter, cut the dough into 3 or 4 large pieces. The shape doesn't matter. Gather, reroll, and cut the scraps as you can. Repeat with the second portion of dough.

TO FILL THE POCKETS

Step 7
Spread about 1 tablespoon of pizza sauce in the middle of each piece. Evenly divide the salami, ham, pepperoni, and cheese between the dough pieces.

Step 8
Gently lift one edge of each piece and fold it over the filling to create a tube. Dip your finger in the egg wash and seal the seam. Push down the edges and seal both ends with some of the egg wash as well. (Reserve the remaining egg wash.) Using the tines of a fork, crimp the edges and transfer the stromboli pockets to the prepared baking sheet. Cover with plastic wrap and let them rest and rise for 30 to 60

minutes.

Step 9

Preheat the oven to 450°F.

Step 10

Using a pastry brush, brush each stromboli pocket with the reserved egg wash. Bake for 15 to 20 minutes, or until golden brown.

Step 11

Let the pockets cool on the baking sheet for 5 minutes and serve. Refrigerate leftovers, covered, for up to 2 days. Reheat to serve.

Sicilian Deep-Dish Pizza

MAKES 1 (9-BY-13-INCH) PIZZA

Prep time: 1 hour 15 minutes
Cook time: 35 minutes

Ingredients:

FOR THE CRUST

- 437 grams Bread Flour Blend
- 1 (7-gram) packet instant (fast-acting) yeast
- 1 tablespoon xanthan gum
- 1 tablespoon salt
- 1 teaspoon cane sugar or granulated sugar
- 1½ cups warm (100° to 110°F) water
- 2 tablespoons extra-virgin olive oil, plus more for the pan and fingertips

FOR THE TOPPING

- 8 slices deli mozzarella cheese or nondairy alternative
- ½ cup gluten-free pizza sauce
- 1 (4-ounce) package sliced gluten-free pepperoni
- 1 ounce Parmesan cheese or nondairy alternative, grated

Directions:

TO MAKE THE CRUST

Step 1

In a large bowl, whisk the flour, yeast, xanthan gum, salt, and sugar to combine. Add the warm water and oil. Using a handheld electric mixer fitted with the dough attachment, mix on medium-high speed until a dough forms.

Step 2

Using a pastry brush (a paper towel is too absorbent and will soak up the oil), generously coat a 9-by-13-inch baking dish with oil, coating the bottom and sides. This will create a crispy crust.

Step 3

Oil your fingertips and transfer the dough into the prepared pan. Using your fingers, spread the dough evenly in the pan so it touches all the edges. Cover the dough with plastic wrap and a clean kitchen towel and let it rest for at least 1 hour.

TO MAKE THE TOPPING

Step 4

Preheat the oven to 450°F.

Step 5

Unwrap the pan and arrange the cheese slices on the dough, leaving a ½-inch border.

Step 6

Pour the pizza sauce in the center of the dough and use the back of a spoon to spread it all around. Add the pepperoni, overlapping, leaving a ½-inch border around the pizza, and sprinkle with Parmesan.

Step 7

Bake for 35 minutes, or until crisp.

Step 8

Run a butter knife along the edges of the pizza to loosen it from the pan. The pizza should come out easily. Cut and serve. Refrigerate leftovers, covered, for up to 2 days.

Everything Bagels

MAKES 8 BAGELS

Prep time: 1 hour 45 minutes
Cook time: 35 minutes

Ingredients:

FOR THE BAGELS

- 375 grams Bread Flour Blend , plus 32 grams
- 1 tablespoon light brown sugar
- 1 tablespoon xanthan gum
- 2 teaspoons baking powder
- 2 teaspoons salt
- 1 teaspoon cane sugar or granulated sugar
- 1 (7-gram) packet instant (fast-acting) yeast
- 1½ cups warm (100° to 110°F) water
- 1 large egg, beaten
- 1 tablespoon honey
- ½ teaspoon apple cider vinegar
- 1 tablespoon olive oil

FOR THE WATER BATH

- ¼ cup honey

FOR THE TOPPING

- 4 teaspoons dried minced garlic
- 4 teaspoons dried minced onion
- 4 teaspoons sesame seeds
- 2 teaspoons poppy seeds
- 2 teaspoons coarse sea salt
- ½ teaspoon freshly ground black pepper
- 1 large egg

Directions:

TO MAKE THE BAGELS

Step 1

Place two sheets of parchment paper on a work surface and place the 32 grams of flour in a corner. Dust a little flour onto one piece of parchment and save the rest.

Step 2

Line 2 baking sheets with parchment paper or silicone baking mats. Take an additional piece of parchment and fold it into eighths. Cut out 8 squares and place them on top of the prepared baking sheets.

Step 3

In a medium bowl, whisk the flour, brown sugar, xanthan gum, baking powder, and salt to combine.

Step 4

In a large bowl, combine the cane sugar, yeast, and 1 cup of warm water. Give it a quick stir and let sit for 5 minutes.

Step 5

Add the beaten egg, remaining ½ cup of warm water, honey, and vinegar. Stir again until combined. Using a handheld electric mixer fitted with the dough hook, add half the flour and mix on low speed to combine. Add the remaining flour and mix to form a dough. The dough will be sticky.

Step 6

Pour the oil into a small dish and dip your fingertips into it. Transfer the dough to the floured work surface. Add some of the remaining 32 grams of flour a little at a time to the dough. If the dough sticks to your fingers, dip them in oil. Repeat this process until the dough is not as sticky. Divide the dough into 8 portions.

Step 7

Roll each dough portion into a ball. Poke a hole through the middle with your finger and smooth the tops. Continue to dip your fingers in the oil if necessary but do not flood the dough with oil. Place each bagel on a parchment square. Cover loosely with plastic wrap and let the dough rest and rise for at least 1 hour.

Step 8

Position an oven rack in the lower third of the oven and preheat the oven to 425°F.

TO MAKE THE WATER BATH

Step 9

In a medium saucepan, stir together 2 quarts of water and honey. Bring to a boil over medium-high heat.

Step 10

Working in batches of 2 to 4 bagels, making sure they have room to move and float, pick each up using the parchment square and carefully drop into the boiling water. Cook for 1 minute, flip and cook for 1 minute more. Once finished, gently and carefully smooth the tops and fix the shape of each with your fingers. Transfer to a wire rack and repeat with the remaining bagels.

TO MAKE THE TOPPING

Step 11

In a shallow bowl, stir together the garlic, onion, sesame seeds, poppy seeds, coarse sea salt, and pepper.

Step 12

In a small bowl, whisk the egg with 1 tablespoon water to create an egg wash. Using a pastry brush, brush the egg wash over the top and sides of each bagel. Dip each coated bagel in the spice topping, turning to coat all sides. Transfer to the prepared baking sheets, 4 bagels per sheet.

Step 13

Bake for 25 to 30 minutes until golden brown.

Step 14

Let the bagels cool for 10 minutes on the baking sheet, then transfer them to a wire rack to cool completely. Tightly wrap and store leftovers in an airtight container at room temperature for up to 3 days or freeze for up to 1 month.

Soft Pretzels

MAKES 4 PRETZELS

Prep time: 2 hours 20 minutes
Cook time: 30 minutes

Ingredients:

- 62 grams All-Purpose Flour Blend , plus more for dusting
- 190 grams Bread Flour Blend
- 1 (7-gram) packet instant (fast-acting) yeast
- 1 tablespoon light brown sugar
- 1½ teaspoons xanthan gum
- 1 teaspoon salt
- 2 large eggs, divided
- ¼ cup sparkling water
- ½ teaspoon apple cider vinegar
- ½ cup warm (100° to 110°F) whole milk or coconut milk beverage
- 1½ teaspoons olive oil
- 2 tablespoons baking soda
- Coarse sea salt

Directions:

Step 1

Line a baking sheet with parchment paper. Place another large sheet of parchment on a clean work surface and dust it with all-purpose flour.

Step 2

In a medium bowl, whisk the all-purpose flour, bread flour, yeast, brown sugar, xanthan gum, and salt to combine.

Step 3

In a large bowl, using a handheld electric mixer, beat 1 egg, the sparkling water, and vinegar. Change to a dough hook and add the flour mixture, mixing on low speed. Add the warm milk and mix to form a dough.

Step 4

Transfer the dough to the floured work surface and dust it with flour to prevent sticking. Shape the dough into an 8-inch log. Cut the log into 4 (2-inch) portions.

Step 5

Pour the oil into a small bowl. Dip your fingertips into the oil and, using your hands, roll one portion into a rope about 12 to 14 inches long. Shape it into a pretzel by bringing the two ends toward you to form a horseshoe shape. Wrap one end over the other and bring the bottom piece around the top piece to form a twist (the ends should still be separate). Bring the ends to the dough ring and press them in to secure. Place on the prepared baking sheet. Repeat with the remaining portions. Cover loosely with plastic wrap and let them rest for at least 2 hours.

Step 6

Preheat the oven to 425°F.

Step 7

In a small saucepan, combine 3 cups water and the baking soda and bring to a boil. Use your finger to smooth out any holes or lumps that have appeared on the dough, and make sure the ends are sealed. One at a time, place each pretzel in the boiling water, front-side down. Boil for 30 seconds per side. The pretzels are delicate, so handle them using 2 forks or a slotted spatula. Transfer the boiled pretzel to the prepared baking sheet.

Step 8

In a small bowl, whisk the remaining egg with 1 tablespoon water to create an egg wash. Using a pastry brush, brush a light layer of egg wash on each pretzel. Sprinkle coarse sea salt over the top.

Step 9

Bake for 20 minutes until the pretzels are golden brown.

Step 10

Let the pretezels cool for 5 minutes on the baking sheet and serve warm, or transfer to a wire rack to cool completely. The pretzels are best eaten the same day.

Skillet Cherry Cobbler

MAKES 1 (12-INCH) COBBLER

Prep time: 20 minutes

Cook time: 45 minutes

Ingredients:

FOR THE SIMPLE SYRUP

- 100 grams cane sugar or granulated sugar

FOR THE FILLING

- 100 grams cane sugar or granulated sugar
- 32 grams All-Purpose Flour Blend
- ¼ teaspoon xanthan gum
- ¼ teaspoon ground cinnamon
- ¼ teaspoon ground nutmeg
- ¼ teaspoon salt
- 1,350 grams frozen cherries
- 1 teaspoon vanilla extract

FOR THE TOPPING

- 190 grams All-Purpose Flour Blend
- 100 grams cane sugar or granulated sugar
- 1½ teaspoons baking powder
- ½ teaspoon xanthan gum
- ¼ teaspoon baking soda
- ¼ teaspoon salt
- ¾ cup whole milk or coconut milk beverage
- 4 tablespoons butter or nondairy alternative, melted
- ½ teaspoon apple cider vinegar
- 2 tablespoons raw turbinado sugar

Directions:

Step 1

Preheat the oven to 425°F.

TO MAKE THE SIMPLE SYRUP

Step 2

In a small saucepan, stir together the cane sugar and ½ cup water. Cook over medium-high heat, stirring until the sugar dissolves, then bring to a boil. Boil for 5 minutes. Transfer to a heatproof bowl to cool.

TO MAKE THE FILLING

Step 3

In a large bowl, whisk the cane sugar, flour, xanthan gum, cinnamon, nutmeg, and salt to combine. Add the frozen cherries and stir to coat. Add the simple syrup and vanilla. Mix to combine.

TO MAKE THE TOPPING

Step 4

In a medium bowl, whisk the flour, cane sugar, baking powder, xanthan gum, baking soda, and salt to combine. Using a spatula, mix in the milk, melted butter, and vinegar until just combined.

Step 5

Pour the sugar-coated cherries into a 12-inch cast-iron skillet and spread them evenly.

Step 6

Using a 1-inch ice cream scoop, drop portions of the topping onto the filling, spacing them about ½ inch apart. Using a spatula, spread the topping over the entire skillet, covering the cherries. Sprinkle the top with the turbinado sugar.

Step 7

Bake for 30 to 35 minutes, or until the topping is golden brown and the filling is thick and glossy.

Step 8

Let the cobbler cool for about 10 minutes before serving warm. Refrigerate leftovers in an airtight container for up to 3 days.

Very Berry Cobbler

MAKES 1 (9-BY-13-INCH) COBBLER

Prep time: 20 minutes

Cook time: 55 minutes

Ingredients:

Shortening, for preparing the pan

FOR THE FILLING

- 2 tablespoons All-Purpose Flour Blend
- ¼ teaspoon xanthan gum
- 50 grams cane sugar or granulated sugar
- 2 teaspoons fresh lemon juice
- 2 teaspoons vanilla extract
- 200 grams blueberries
- 230 grams blackberries
- 250 grams raspberries

FOR THE TOPPING

- 156 grams All-Purpose Flour Blend , plus more for dusting

- ½ teaspoon xanthan gum
- 1 teaspoon baking powder
- ¼ teaspoon salt
- 50 grams cane sugar or granulated sugar
- 67 grams shortening
- 1 large egg yolk
- ¼ cup buttermilk, plus 2 tablespoons, or ¼ cup plus 2 tablespoons coconut milk beverage plus 2 teaspoons apple cider vinegar (see here)
- Raw turbinado sugar, for sprinkling

Directions:

Step 1

Preheat the oven to 350°F. Grease a 9-by-13-inch pan with shortening.

TO MAKE THE FILLING

Step 2

In a small bowl, whisk the flour and xanthan gum to combine. Add the sugar, lemon juice, and vanilla and mix well. If it's clumpy, don't worry.

Step 3

In a large bowl, combine the blueberries, blackberries, and raspberries. Pour the flour mixture on top and use a spatula to gently fold into the berries. Transfer the mixed berries to the prepared pan, cover with aluminum foil, and refrigerate until needed.

TO MAKE THE TOPPING

Step 4

Place two sheets of parchment paper on a work surface and dust them with flour.

Step 5

In a medium bowl, whisk the flour and xanthan gum to combine. Add the baking powder, salt, and sugar. Whisk well.

Step 6

Using a pastry cutter, cut the shortening into the flour mixture until it forms coarse crumbs. Add the egg yolk and ¼ cup of buttermilk. Form the dough by hand. Transfer it to the flour-dusted work surface. Pat the dough into a flat rectangle, dusting the top with a little bit of flour. Place the second sheet of parchment over the top. Using a rolling pin, flatten the dough to about the size of your baking pan.

Step 7

Remove the berries from the refrigerator. Lift the top layer of parchment, place your right hand underneath the bottom layer of parchment paper and your left hand on top of the dough, and gently flip the dough over and on top of the berries. Peel off the remaining piece of parchment and adjust the edges of the dough to fit nicely over the berries in your pan.

Step 8

Using a pastry brush, brush the dough with the remaining 2 tablespoons of buttermilk. Sprinkle with turbinado sugar.

Step 9

Bake for 45 to 55 minutes, or until the top is golden.

Step 10

Let the cobbler cool on a wire rack for 10 minutes before serving. Refrigerate leftovers, covered, for up to 5 days.

Peach Cobbler

MAKES 1 (11-BY-7-INCH) COBBLER

Prep time: 20 minutes

Cook time: 40 minutes

Ingredients:

- Shortening, for preparing the pan

FOR THE FILLING

- 1,000 grams sliced peeled peaches (about 10 peaches)
- 50 grams light brown sugar
- 2 tablespoons All-Purpose Flour Blend
- ¼ teaspoon xanthan gum

FOR THE TOPPING

- 250 grams All-Purpose Flour Blend
- 1 tablespoon baking powder
- 1 teaspoon xanthan gum
- 1 teaspoon ground cinnamon
- ¼ teaspoon salt
- ½ cup whole milk or coconut milk beverage
- 1 large egg
- 1 teaspoon apple cider vinegar
- 8 tablespoons (1 stick) cold butter or nondairy alternative
- 2 tablespoons raw turbinado sugar

Directions:

Step 1

Preheat the oven to 425°F. Grease an 11-by-7-inch baking dish or a 9-by-9-inch pan with shortening.

TO MAKE THE FILLING

Step 2

Place the peaches in a large bowl and pour the brown sugar over them.

Step 3

In a small bowl, whisk the flour and xanthan gum to combine and add it to the peaches. Stir to combine everything.

TO MAKE THE TOPPING

Step 4

In a medium bowl, whisk the flour, baking powder, xanthan gum, cinnamon, and salt to combine.

Step 5

In a small bowl, whisk the milk, egg, and vinegar.

Step 6

Using a pastry cutter, cut the cold butter into pieces and mix it into the flour mixture. Drizzle in the egg mixture and, using a spatula, stir just until combined. It should be lumpy.

Step 7

Pour the peaches into the prepared baking dish.

Step 8

Using a 1-inch ice cream scoop, drop chunks of the topping over the peaches, spacing them about ½ inch apart. Using a spatula, spread the topping over the entire pan. Sprinkle the turbinado sugar evenly over the top. Loosely cover the pan with aluminum foil.

Step 9

Bake for 30 minutes. Remove the foil and bake for 10 minutes more until golden.

Step 10

Serve warm or at room temperature. Refrigerate leftovers, covered, for up to 3 days.

Vanilla Cupcakes

MAKES 12 CUPCAKES

Prep time: 15 minutes

Cook time: 20 minutes

Ingredients:

FOR THE CUPCAKES

- 190 grams All-Purpose Flour Blend
- 1 teaspoon baking powder
- ½ teaspoon xanthan gum
- ¼ teaspoon baking soda
- ¼ teaspoon salt
- 3 large egg whites
- 200 grams cane sugar or granulated sugar
- ½ cup avocado oil or canola oil
- ¼ cup whole milk or coconut milk beverage
- 1 tablespoon vanilla extract

FOR THE FROSTING

- 134 grams shortening
- 1 teaspoon vanilla extract
- 480 grams powdered sugar, plus more as needed

Directions:

TO MAKE THE CUPCAKES

Step 1

Preheat the oven to 350°F. Line a 12-cup muffin tin with cupcake liners.

Step 2

In a small bowl, whisk the flour, baking powder, xanthan gum, baking soda, and salt to combine.

Step 3

In a large bowl, using a handheld electric mixer, whip the egg whites until they form a soft peak. Add the cane sugar, oil, milk, and vanilla. Mix well. Add the flour mixture and mix until combined.

Step 4

Evenly divide the batter between the prepared muffin cups, filling them three-quarters full.

Step 5

Bake for 18 to 20 minutes, or until a toothpick inserted into the center of a cupcake comes out clean.

Step 6

Let the cupcakes cool in the pan for 10 minutes, then transfer them to a wire rack to cool completely.

TO MAKE THE FROSTING

Step 7

While the cupcakes are cooling, in a large bowl, using a handheld electric mixer on medium speed, cream together the shortening and vanilla until smooth.

Step 8

Add the powdered sugar and mix on low speed until smooth and creamy, adding 1 tablespoon of water at a time until you get the desired consistency. If the frosting is too thick, add 1 tablespoon more of water; if it is too thin, add 1 tablespoon of powdered sugar.

Step 9

Fill a piping bag fitted your desired tip with the frosting and decorate each cupcake as desired. Keep covered at room temperature for up to 4 days.

Pumpkin Pie Cupcakes

MAKES 12 CUPCAKES
Prep time: 15 minutes
Cook time: 30 minutes

Ingredients:

FOR THE CUPCAKES

- 125 grams All-Purpose Flour Blend
- 2 teaspoons pumpkin pie spice
- 1 teaspoon ground cinnamon
- ½ teaspoon xanthan gum
- ¼ teaspoon ground cloves
- ¼ teaspoon baking powder
- ¼ teaspoon baking soda
- ¼ teaspoon salt
- 1 (7.4-ounce) can sweetened condensed coconut milk
- 150 grams cane sugar or granulated sugar
- 2 large eggs
- 1 (15-ounce) can pumpkin puree

FOR THE COCONUT WHIPPED CREAM

- 1 (14-ounce) can coconut cream, chilled overnight
- 2 tablespoons powdered sugar

Directions:

TO MAKE THE CUPCAKES

Step 1

Preheat the oven to 350°F. Line a 12-cup muffin tin with cupcake liners.

Step 2

In a small bowl, whisk the flour, pumpkin pie spice, cinnamon, xanthan gum, cloves, baking powder, baking soda, and salt to combine.

Step 3

In a large bowl, using a spatula, mix the condensed coconut milk and cane sugar. Stir all the clumps out of the milk. Add the eggs and mix well. Add the pumpkin puree and the flour mixture. Stir just until combined. Do not overmix.

Step 4

Scoop the batter evenly into the prepared muffin cups.

Step 5

Bake for 28 to 30 minutes, or until a toothpick inserted into the center of a cupcake comes out clean.

Step 6

Let the cupcakes cool in the pan for 30 minutes.

Gingerbread Cupcakes

MAKES 12 CUPCAKES

Prep time: 25 minutes

Cook time: 22 minutes

Ingredients:

FOR THE CUPCAKES

- 167 grams All-Purpose Flour Blend
- 2 tablespoons arrowroot
- 1½ teaspoons ground cinnamon
- ½ teaspoon xanthan gum
- ½ teaspoon baking powder
- ½ teaspoon baking soda
- ½ teaspoon ground ginger
- ½ teaspoon ground nutmeg
- ½ teaspoon ground cloves
- ¼ teaspoon salt
- ½ cup avocado oil or canola oil
- 100 grams light brown sugar
- ½ cup whole milk or coconut milk beverage
- ½ cup maple syrup
- 1 large egg
- 1 teaspoon vanilla extract
- ½ teaspoon apple cider vinegar

FOR THE CREAM CHEESE FROSTING

- 102 grams shortening
- 4 ounces cream cheese or nondairy alternative
- 480 grams powdered sugar
- 1 teaspoon vanilla extract
- 4 tablespoons whole milk or coconut milk beverage

Directions:

TO MAKE THE CUPCAKES

Step 1

Preheat the oven to 350°F. Line a 12-cup muffin tin with cupcake liners.

Step 2

In a medium bowl, whisk the flour, arrowroot, cinnamon, xanthan gum, baking powder, baking soda, ginger, nutmeg, cloves, and salt to combine.

Step 3

In a large bowl, using a handheld electric mixer, beat the oil and brown sugar to blend. Add the milk, maple syrup, egg, vanilla, and vinegar. Mix well. Beat in the flour mixture in two additions, mixing to combine, and stopping to scrape down the bowl as needed, making sure there are no brown sugar clumps.

Step 4

Evenly divide the batter between the prepared muffin cups, filling them two-thirds full.

Step 5

Bake for 20 to 22 minutes, or until a toothpick inserted into the center of a cupcake comes out clean.

Step 6

Let the cupcakes cool in the pan for at least 10 minutes, then transfer to a wire rack to cool completely.

TO MAKE THE CREAM CHEESE FROSTING

Step 7

In a large bowl, using a handheld electric mixer on medium speed, cream together the shortening and cream cheese. Add the powdered sugar and vanilla. Mix as you add the milk by the tablespoon until smooth and creamy.

Step 8

Frost the cupcakes. Refrigerate leftovers, covered, for up to 5 days.

Death-by-Chocolate Cake

MAKES 1 (9-INCH) TWO-LAYER FROSTED CAKE

Prep time: 35 minutes
Cook time: 28 minutes

Ingredients:

FOR THE CAKE
- Shortening, for preparing the pans
- 157 grams All-Purpose Flour Blend, plus more for dusting
- 75 grams unsweetened natural cocoa powder
- 62 grams arrowroot
- 2 teaspoons ground espresso
- 2 teaspoons baking soda
- 1 teaspoon baking powder
- 1 teaspoon xanthan gum
- 1 teaspoon salt
- 350 grams cane sugar or granulated sugar
- 1 cup avocado oil or canola oil
- 2 large eggs
- 1 cup whole milk or coconut milk beverage
- 60 grams vanilla Greek yogurt or nondairy alternative
- 1 shot brewed espresso, cooled (optional)
- 2 tablespoons vanilla extract

- 1 teaspoon apple cider vinegar

FOR THE CHOCOLATE BUTTERCREAM FROSTING

- 136 grams shortening
- 720 grams powdered sugar
- 75 grams unsweetened natural cocoa powder
- 2 teaspoons vanilla extract
- 6 tablespoons whole milk or coconut milk beverage

Directions:

TO MAKE THE CAKE

Step 1

Preheat the oven to 350°F. Grease two 9-inch springform pans with shortening. Sprinkle a little flour inside and tap the pans to spread the flour evenly around each pan.

Step 2

In a medium bowl, whisk the flour, cocoa powder, arrowroot, ground espresso, baking soda, baking powder, xanthan gum, and salt to combine.

Step 3

In a large bowl, using a whisk or handheld electric mixer, beat the sugar, oil, eggs, milk, yogurt, brewed espresso (if using), vanilla, and vinegar until well mixed, stopping to scrape down the bowl as needed. Slowly add the flour mixture and mix until combined.

Step 4

Evenly divide the batter between the prepared pans.

Step 5

Bake for 25 to 28 minutes, or until a toothpick inserted into the center of a cake comes out clean.

Step 6

Let the cakes cool in the pans for at least 15 minutes. Release the clamp from each pan and remove the sides. Transfer the cakes and plates to a wire rack to cool completely.

Step 7

Using a large serrated knife, cut off the thin domed layer from the top of each cake. Creating a flat surface will help the cakes stack well.

TO MAKE THE CHOCOLATE BUTTERCREAM FROSTING

Step 8

In a large bowl, using a handheld electric mixer, beat the shortening until smooth and creamy. Add the powdered sugar, cocoa powder, and vanilla. Mix, while slowly adding the milk, until smooth and creamy.

Step 9

Frost the cake layers and outside of the cake as desired. Refrigerate leftovers, covered, for up to 5 days.

Super Moist Cream Cheese Pound Cake

MAKES 1 TUBE CAKE

Prep time: 20 minutes
Cook time: 1 hour 20 minutes

Ingredients:

- Shortening, for preparing the pan
- 375 grams All-Purpose Flour Blend

- 3 tablespoons arrowroot
- 1 teaspoon xanthan gum
- ½ teaspoon baking powder
- ¼ teaspoon salt
- 24 tablespoons (3 sticks) butter or nondairy alternative
- 1 (8-ounce) package cream cheese or nondairy alternative
- 500 grams cane sugar or granulated sugar
- 80 grams vanilla Greek yogurt or nondairy alternative
- 6 large eggs, beaten
- 2 teaspoons vanilla extract

Directions:

Step 1

Preheat the oven to 325°F. Grease a 10- to 12-cup Bundt pan with shortening.

Step 2

In a medium bowl, whisk the flour, arrowroot, xanthan gum, baking powder, and salt to combine.

Step 3

In a large bowl, using a handheld electric mixer on medium speed, cream together the butter and cream cheese, stopping to scrape down the bowl as needed. Add the sugar and mix well. Add the yogurt, beaten eggs, and vanilla. Mix until combined.

Step 4

Add the flour mixture to the wet ingredients and mix just until combined. Do not overmix.

Step 5

Pour the batter into the prepared Bundt pan and tap the pan on the counter to remove any air bubbles.

Step 6

Bake for 1 hour 15 minutes to 1 hour 20 minutes, or until a toothpick inserted into the center of the pound cake comes out clean.

Step 7

Let the cake cool completely in the pan. This may take 1 to 2 hours. Invert the cake over a wire rack and remove it from the pan. Keep covered at room temperature, or refrigerate, for up to 5 days.

Buttery Mini Tarts

MAKES 12 MINI TARTS

Prep time: about 1 hour, plus 1 hour to chill
Cook time: 25 minutes

Ingredients:

FOR THE FILLING

- 32 grams All-Purpose Flour Blend
- ¼ teaspoon xanthan gum
- 4 large egg yolks
- 100 grams cane sugar or granulated sugar
- 1 teaspoon vanilla extract
- ¾ cup whole milk or coconut milk beverage
- ¾ cup heavy cream or nondairy alternative

- Grated zest of 1 lemon

FOR THE TARTS
- 8 tablespoons (1 stick) cold butter or nondairy alternative
- Shortening, for preparing the pans
- 125 grams <u>All-Purpose Flour Blend</u> , plus more for dusting
- 32 grams brown rice flour
- 32 grams sorghum flour
- 60 grams powdered sugar
- 1 teaspoon xanthan gum
- ¼ teaspoon salt
- 1 large egg
- ½ teaspoon apple cider vinegar
- ½ teaspoon vanilla extract

Directions:

TO MAKE THE FILLING

Step 1

In a small bowl, whisk the flour and xanthan gum to combine.

Step 2

In a small bowl, whisk the egg yolks, sugar, and vanilla to blend.

Step 3

In a small saucepan, combine the milk, cream, and lemon zest. Heat over medium heat until hot but do not boil.

Step 4

Whisk the flour mixture into the egg mixture. Then, whisking constantly, use a ladle to slowly add a small and steady stream of the warm cream mixture to the flour/egg mixture. Keep whisking so the egg yolks do not scramble. Repeat with one more ladle of cream mixture.

Step 5

Return the pan to medium heat and cook, stirring constantly, for 5 to 7 minutes, or until thickened. Transfer to a glass bowl and cover with plastic wrap, pushing the plastic down so it touches the filling. Refrigerate for at least 1 hour or overnight.

TO MAKE THE TARTS

Step 6

Cut the butter into pieces and put it in the freezer for 30 minutes.

Step 7

Grease 12 mini tart molds or a 12-well mini tart pan with shortening. Place two sheets of parchment paper on a work surface and dust them with flour.

Step 8

In a small bowl, whisk the all-purpose flour, rice flour, sorghum flour, powdered sugar, xanthan gum, and salt to combine.

Step 9

In a small bowl, whisk the egg, vinegar, and vanilla to blend.

Step 10

Using a pastry cutter, cut the butter into the flour mixture until crumbs form. Add the egg mixture and mix to form the dough.

Step 11

Transfer the dough to the floured work surface. Dust the top of the dough with a little flour and place it between the two sheets of parchment. Roll the dough to ⅛ inch thick. Using a 3-inch round cookie cutter, cut out 12 rounds. Using a spatula, transfer the rounds to the prepared molds and press them firmly into the molds. Transfer the molds to a baking sheet and chill for 1 hour.

Step 12

Preheat the oven to 400°F.

Step 13

Cut twelve 2-by-2-inch pieces of parchment paper to fit into the tarts and line the tarts with them. Fill each tart with dried beans or mini pie weights.

Step 14

Bake for 15 minutes. Carefully remove the parchment paper and weights. Prick holes all over the bottoms of the tarts with a fork. Bake for 10 to 12 minutes more, or until firm and golden brown. Transfer to a wire rack to cool.

Step 15

Fill the cooled tarts with the filling and enjoy. Refrigerate leftovers, covered, for up to 3 days.

Vanilla Donuts

MAKES 12 DONUTS

Prep time: 15 minutes
Cook time: 16 minutes

Ingredients:

- Shortening, for preparing the pans
- 282 grams All-Purpose Flour Blend
- 150 grams cane sugar or granulated sugar
- 2 teaspoons baking powder
- 1 teaspoon salt
- ½ teaspoon xanthan gum
- ½ teaspoon ground cinnamon
- 1 cup buttermilk, or 1 cup coconut milk beverage plus 1 tablespoon apple cider vinegar (see here)
- ½ cup avocado oil or canola oil, plus more for frying
- 2 large eggs
- 2 teaspoons vanilla extract
- Glaze (from Cinnamon Roll Pancakes)

Directions:

Step 1

Preheat the oven to 425°F. Grease two 6-well donut pans with shortening.

Step 2

In a small bowl, whisk the flour, sugar, baking powder, salt, xanthan gum, and cinnamon to combine.

Step 3

In a large bowl, using a handheld electric mixer, beat the buttermilk, oil, eggs, and vanilla. Add the flour mixture to the egg mixture and beat until combined.

Step 4

Transfer the batter to a piping or plastic bag and cut the tip. Divide the batter evenly between the prepared wells of the donut pans. Jiggle each pan to smooth any ribbons in the batter.

Step 5

Bake for 9 minutes, then (without opening the oven) reduce the temperature to 350°F and bake for 5 to 7 minutes more, or until a toothpick inserted into a donut comes out clean.

Step 6

Let the donuts cool in the pans for 10 minutes, then transfer to a wire rack to cool completely.

Step 7

Place a skillet over medium heat and add about ⅛ inch of oil. You'll know the oil is ready when a drop of water sizzles in it. Place 2 or 3 donuts facedown (lighter-side down) in the oil and flash-fry for 2 to 3 minutes, or until the donuts sizzle and pick up a little color. Watch closely to prevent burning. Flip and flash-fry the other side for 1 to 2 minutes. Return the donuts to the rack to cool.

Step 8

Repeat with the remaining donuts. As the oil gets hotter, the donuts will need less time. Be careful not to burn them. Add more oil, as needed.

Step 9

Dip each donut into the glaze and let set completely. These are best served the same day but can be kept covered at room temperature for up to 3 days. Humidity can make the glaze melt.

Beignets

MAKES 15 BEIGNETS

Prep time: 30 minutes
Cook time: 15 minutes

Ingredients:

- 125 grams All-Purpose Flour Blend
- 1 teaspoon baking powder
- ½ teaspoon xanthan gum
- ¼ teaspoon ground cinnamon
- ¼ teaspoon salt
- 150 grams cane sugar or granulated sugar
- 2 large eggs, separated
- 1 tablespoon butter or nondairy alternative, melted
- 1 teaspoon vanilla extract
- ½ teaspoon apple cider vinegar
- Oil or shortening, for frying
- 120 grams powdered sugar

Directions:

Step 1

In a medium bowl, whisk the flour, baking powder, xanthan gum, cinnamon, and salt to combine.

Step 2

In a medium bowl, using a handheld electric mixer, beat the cane sugar, egg yolks, ¼ cup water, melted butter, vanilla, and vinegar.

Step 3

In another medium bowl, using a handheld electric mixer, whip the egg whites until soft peaks form.

Step 4

Using a spatula, add the egg yolk mixture to the flour mixture and mix until combined. Still using a spatula, stir in half the whipped egg whites, then add the remaining egg whites and stir until combined again.

Step 5

Place a paper towel over a wire rack and place the rack on a baking sheet. Pour about 3 inches of oil into a large, deep heavy-bottomed pan and heat to 350°F over medium heat.

Step 6

Coat the inside of a 1-inch ice cream scoop with a little oil. Scoop balls of dough into the hot oil. Fry for 2 to 3 minutes until golden brown, turning so all sides gain color. Place them on the paper towel to drain. Repeat with the remaining dough.

Step 7

Generously dust the beignets with powdered sugar before serving. Keep leftovers covered at room temperature for up to 3 days.

Apple Cider Cinnamon Donuts

MAKES 12 DONUTS

Prep time: 25 minutes

Cook time: 20 minutes

Ingredients:

FOR THE DONUTS

- 1½ cups apple cider
- Shortening, for preparing the pans
- 313 grams All-Purpose Flour Blend
- 1 teaspoon baking soda
- 1 teaspoon baking powder
- 1 teaspoon ground cinnamon
- 1 teaspoon gluten-free apple pie spice
- ½ teaspoon xanthan gum
- ¼ teaspoon salt
- 100 grams light brown sugar
- 100 grams cane sugar or granulated sugar
- 120 grams unsweetened applesauce
- 2 tablespoons butter or nondairy alternative, melted
- 1 large egg
- 1 teaspoon vanilla extract
- Oil or shortening, for frying

FOR THE TOPPING

- 5 tablespoons butter or nondairy alternative, melted
- 200 grams cane sugar or granulated sugar
- 1 teaspoon ground cinnamon
- 1 teaspoon gluten-free apple pie spice

Directions:
TO MAKE THE DONUTS
Step 1

In a small saucepan, cook the apple cider over medium, stirring constantly, for about 10 minutes, or until reduced by half. Remove from the heat and let the cider cool to room temperature.

Step 2

Preheat the oven to 350°F. Grease two 6-well donut pans with shortening.

Step 3

In a medium bowl, whisk the flour, baking soda, baking powder, cinnamon, apple pie spice, xanthan gum, and salt to combine.

Step 4

In a large bowl, using a handheld electric mixer, beat the brown sugar, cane sugar, applesauce, melted butter, egg, and vanilla until combined.

Step 5

Using a spatula, stir in half the flour mixture, followed by half the reduced cider. Stir in the remaining flour and apple cider until combined. Transfer the batter to a piping bag or plastic bag. Cut the tip and evenly fill the prepared donut wells with batter.

Step 6

Bake for 10 to 11 minutes, or until a toothpick inserted into the center of a donut comes out clean.

Step 7

Let the donuts cool in the pans for 10 minutes, then carefully remove them from the pan and transfer to a wire rack to cool completely.

Step 8

In a skillet, heat about ⅛ inch of oil over medium heat. You'll know the oil is ready when a drop of water sizzles in it. Place 2 or 3 donuts facedown (lighter-side down) in the oil and flash-fry for 2 to 3 minutes, or until the donuts sizzle and pick up a little color. Watch closely to prevent burning. Flip and flash-fry the other side for 1 to 2 minutes. Transfer the donuts back to the rack to cool.

Step 9

Repeat with the remaining donuts. As the oil gets hotter, the donuts will need less time. Be careful not to burn them. Add more oil, as needed.

TO MAKE THE TOPPING
Step 10

Place the melted butter in a small bowl.

Step 11

In another small bowl, stir together the sugar, cinnamon, and apple pie spice.

Step 12

Using a pastry brush, coat the top and bottom of each donut with melted butter, then dip it in the apple cinnamon topping to cover it completely. Keep covered at room temperature for up to 3 days.

Churros

MAKES 20 CHURROS
Prep time: 15 minutes
Cook time: 15 minutes

Ingredients:
- 2 teaspoons ground cinnamon
- 100 grams cane sugar or granulated sugar, plus 2 tablespoons
- 125 grams All-Purpose Flour Blend
- 1 teaspoon salt
- ¼ teaspoon xanthan gum
- 6 tablespoons butter or nondairy alternative
- 2 large eggs
- 1 teaspoon vanilla extract
- Oil or shortening, for frying

Directions:

Step 1

Prepare a piping bag with a 1M star tip and set aside. Place a paper towel on a wire cooling rack and place the rack on a baking sheet.

Step 2

On a large plate, stir together the cinnamon and 100 grams of sugar.

Step 3

In a small bowl, whisk the flour, salt, and xanthan gum to combine.

Step 4

In a medium saucepan, combine the butter, remaining 2 tablespoons of sugar, and 1 cup water. Cook over medium heat, stirring, until the butter and sugar melt. Bring to a soft boil for about 2 minutes, then remove from the heat and stir in the flour mixture. Let the dough cool for 10 minutes.

Step 5

Transfer the churro dough to a large bowl. Using a handheld electric mixer, beat in the eggs, one at a time, until just incorporated. Mix in the vanilla. Fill the piping bag with the batter and lay it flat.

Step 6

Pour 3 inches of oil into a large, deep heavy-bottomed pan and heat to 350°F over medium heat.

Step 7

Holding the piping bag several inches above the oil, pipe a 6-inch rope into the oil, using kitchen shears to cut it off at the tip. Repeat a few more times, depending on the size of your pan. Fry for 4 to 5 minutes, turning, until golden. Using a slotted spoon, transfer the churros to the plate and roll them in the cinnamon sugar. Place them on the prepared rack to cool. Repeat with the remaining batter.

Step 8

Churros are best served warm on the same day they were made.

Garlic Butter Breadsticks

MAKES 8 BREADSTICKS

Prep time: 2 hours 15 minutes
Cook time: 15 minutes

Ingredients:

FOR THE BREADSTICKS

190 grams Bread Flour Blend

2 tablespoons cane sugar or granulated sugar, divided

1 teaspoon salt

1 teaspoon xanthan gum

½ teaspoon baking powder

1½ tablespoons olive oil

¼ teaspoon garlic powder

1 teaspoon instant (fast-acting) yeast

¾ cup warm (100° 110°F) water

½ teaspoon apple cider vinegar

FOR THE GARLIC BUTTER

2 tablespoons butter or nondairy alternative

½ teaspoon garlic powder

Directions:

TO MAKE THE BREADSTICKS

Step 1

Line a baking sheet with parchment paper or a silicone baking mat.

Step 2

In a medium bowl, whisk the flour, 1 tablespoon of sugar, the salt, xanthan gum, and baking powder to combine.

Step 3

In a small bowl, stir together the oil and garlic powder.

Step 4

In a large bowl, stir together the yeast, remaining 1 tablespoon of sugar, and warm water. Let sit for 5 minutes.

Step 5

Add the garlic oil and vinegar and give it a quick stir. Using a handheld electric mixer fitted with the dough attachment, or your clean hands, add half the flour mixture to the wet ingredients and mix on low speed to combine. Add the remaining flour mixture and mix to form a dough. It will be sticky.

Step 6

Transfer the dough to a piping bag or plastic bag and cut the tip to about a 1-inch width. Squeeze the dough into 6-inch ropes onto the prepared baking sheet. Cover loosely with plastic wrap and let the dough rest and rise for at least 2 hours.

TO MAKE THE GARLIC BUTTER

Step 7

In a small saucepan, melt the butter over low heat. Stir in the garlic powder and cook, stirring, until the garlic powder dissolves.

Step 8

Position an oven rack in the lower third of the oven and preheat the oven to 425°F.

Step 9

Using a pastry brush, brush the breadsticks with some of the garlic butter. Reserve the remainder.

Step 10

Bake for 15 minutes, or until slightly golden.

Step 11

Remove from the oven and brush the breadsticks with the reserved garlic butter. Let the breadsticks cool on the baking sheet for 10 minutes.

Step 12

Serve warm or cool. Best served same day. Keep leftovers in an airtight container at room temperature for up to 3 days, or freeze for up to 1 month. Rewarm to serve.

Perfect Skillet Pancakes

MAKES 6 PANCAKES

Prep time: 10 minutes
Cook time: 20 minutes

Ingredients:

- Butter, for greasing the skillet
- 125 grams All-Purpose Flour Blend
- 2 tablespoons cane sugar or granulated sugar
- 1½ teaspoons baking powder
- ½ teaspoon salt
- ¼ teaspoon xanthan gum
- ¼ teaspoon baking soda
- ¾ cup whole milk or coconut milk beverage
- 1 large egg
- 2 tablespoons avocado oil or canola oil
- Maple syrup, for serving

Directions:

Step 1

Heat a skillet over low heat. Cut off a chunk of stick butter long enough to hold on to and have it at the ready.

Step 2

In a medium bowl, whisk the flour, sugar, baking powder, salt, xanthan gum, and baking soda to combine. Add the milk, egg, and oil. Mix to blend. Let the batter sit for 5 minutes.

Step 3

Hold the chunk of butter and use it to grease the skillet, spreading it all around the skillet as you increase the heat to medium. Pour ¼ cup of batter into the skillet. Cook for about 3 minutes, or until bubbles form and begin to pop. Flip the pancake to the other side and cook for 2 to 3 minutes more, until set. The pancakes take less time to cook on the second side. Rub each pancake with butter and watch it melt into the pancake. Repeat with the remaining pancake batter, using more butter to grease the skillet as necessary.

Step 4

Drizzle maple syrup on top to serve. These are best served warm immediately.

Mom's French Toast

MAKES 6 SLICES

Prep time: 15 minutes
Cook time: 25 minutes

Ingredients:

- 100 grams light brown sugar

- 1 teaspoon ground cinnamon
- 8 tablespoons (1 stick) butter or nondairy alternative, melted and slightly cooled
- 2 large eggs, beaten
- 1 cup whole milk or coconut milk beverage
- 2 tablespoons maple syrup, plus more for serving
- 1 tablespoon vanilla extract
- 6 slices gluten-free <u>Sandwich Bread</u>
- Gluten-free cooking spray
- Powdered sugar, for dusting

Directions:

Step 1

In a medium bowl, combine the brown sugar, cinnamon, melted butter, eggs, milk, maple syrup, and vanilla, in that order, and whisk to blend. Pour the mixture into a 9-by-13-inch baking pan. Add the bread slices and let sit for 1 to 2 minutes. Flip and let sit for 1 to 2 minutes more. Be careful not to let them sit too long or the bread will become soggy and break.

Step 2

Heat a skillet over medium heat. Coat the skillet with cooking spray. Place 1 slice of bread in the skillet and cook for about 3 minutes, or until the bottom seems to crisp up. Flip and cook for 2 to 3 minutes more. Repeat with the remaining slices.

Step 3

Dust the toast with powdered sugar and drizzle with maple syrup.

Overnight Waffles

MAKES 8 WAFFLES

Prep time: 10 minutes, plus overnight to chill
Cook time: 20 minutes

Ingredients:

- 250 grams All-Purpose Flour Blend
- 1 tablespoon baking powder
- 1 teaspoon salt
- ½ teaspoon xanthan gum
- ½ teaspoon ground cinnamon
- 1 cup whole milk or coconut milk beverage
- 2 large eggs
- 6 tablespoons maple syrup, plus more for serving
- 4 tablespoons melted butter or nondairy alternative, cooled slightly, plus more for serving
- 1 teaspoon vanilla extract
- ½ teaspoon apple cider vinegar
- Gluten-free cooking spray

Directions:

Step 1

In a medium bowl, whisk the flour, baking powder, salt, xanthan gum, and cinnamon to combine.

Step 2

In a small bowl, whisk the milk, eggs, maple syrup, melted butter, vanilla, and vinegar.

Step 3

Make a small well in the middle of the flour mixture and add the egg mixture. Mix well. Cover the bowl and refrigerate overnight.

Step 4

Preheat a waffle iron according to the manufacturer's instructions. Coat it with cooking spray. Place ¼ cup of batter in the middle of the waffle iron and cook according to the manufacturer's instructions.

Step 5

Top with butter and drizzle with maple syrup.

Glazed Lemon Poppy Seed Loaf

MAKES 1 (9-BY-5-INCH) LOAF

Prep time: 20 minutes

Cook time: about 1 hour

Ingredients:

FOR THE BREAD

- Gluten-free cooking spray
- 375 grams All-Purpose Flour Blend
- 1 tablespoon poppy seeds
- 1½ teaspoons baking powder
- 1½ teaspoons xanthan gum
- ¾ teaspoon salt
- ½ teaspoon baking soda
- 100 grams cane sugar or granulated sugar
- 100 grams light brown sugar
- 3 large eggs
- ½ cup avocado oil or canola oil
- ⅔ cup cold water
- 2 tablespoons grated lemon zest
- 2 tablespoons fresh lemon juice
- 2 teaspoons vanilla extract

FOR THE LEMON GLAZE

- 210 grams powdered sugar
- 2 tablespoons grated lemon zest
- 2 tablespoons fresh lemon juice

Directions:

TO MAKE THE BREAD

Step 1

Preheat the oven to 350°F. Coat a 9-by-5-inch loaf pan with cooking spray or line it with parchment paper.

Step 2

In a medium bowl, whisk the flour, poppy seeds, baking powder, xanthan gum, salt, and baking soda to combine.

Step 3

In a large bowl, using a handheld electric mixer, beat the cane sugar, brown sugar, eggs, oil, cold water, lemon zest, lemon juice, and vanilla for 2 minutes. Add the flour mixture and beat until combined. Do not overmix. Pour the batter into the prepared loaf pan.

Step 4

Bake for 50 to 60 minutes, or until a toothpick inserted into the center of the loaf comes out clean.

Step 5

Let the loaf cool in the pan for 15 minutes, then gently remove the loaf and transfer it to a wire rack to cool completely.

TO MAKE THE LEMON GLAZE

Step 6

While the loaf cools, in a medium bowl, stir together the powdered sugar, lemon zest, and lemon juice until smooth.

Step 7

Pour the glaze over the cooled loaf. Tightly wrap any remaining bread and keep it at room temperature for up to 3 days, or refrigerate for up to 1 week.

Cinnamon Swirl Loaf

MAKES 1 (9-BY-5-INCH) LOAF

Prep time: 20 minutes

Cook time: about 50 minutes

Ingredients:

FOR THE TOPPING

- 1 tablespoon light brown sugar
- 1 tablespoon cane sugar or granulated sugar
- 1 teaspoon ground cinnamon

FOR THE FILLING

- 2 tablespoons butter or nondairy alternative, melted
- 50 grams light brown sugar
- 2 tablespoons All-Purpose Flour Blend
- 1 tablespoon ground cinnamon

FOR THE LOAF

- Gluten-free cooking spray
- 250 grams All-Purpose Flour Blend
- 100 grams cane sugar or granulated sugar
- 100 grams light brown sugar
- 1 teaspoon xanthan gum
- 1 teaspoon baking powder
- ½ teaspoon baking soda
- ¼ teaspoon salt
- 1 cup buttermilk, or 1 cup coconut milk beverage plus 1 tablespoon apple cider vinegar (see here)
- 2 large eggs
- ¼ cup avocado oil or canola oil
- 2 teaspoons vanilla extract

Directions:

TO MAKE THE TOPPING

Step 1

In a small bowl, stir together the brown sugar, cane sugar, and cinnamon until blended.

TO MAKE THE FILLING

Step 2

In another small bowl, stir together the melted butter, brown sugar, flour, and cinnamon until combined.

TO MAKE THE LOAF

Step 3

Preheat the oven to 350°F. Coat a 9-by-5-inch loaf pan with cooking spray or line it with parchment paper.

Step 4

In a medium bowl, whisk the flour, cane sugar, brown sugar, xanthan gum, baking powder, baking soda, and salt to combine.

Step 5

In a large bowl, using a handheld electric mixer, beat the buttermilk, eggs, oil, and vanilla for 2 minutes. Add the flour mixture and beat until combined. Do not overmix.

Step 6

Pour half the batter into the prepared loaf pan. Drizzle the filling evenly on top. Pour the remaining batter over the filling. Using a butter knife, cut an "S" shape down the length of the pan to create the swirl. Finish by sprinkling the topping over the loaf.

Step 7

Bake for 45 to 50 minutes, or until a toothpick inserted into the center of the loaf comes out clean.

Step 8

Let the loaf cool in the pan for 15 minutes, then gently remove it and transfer to a wire rack to cool completely. Keep any remaining slices covered at room temperature for up to 3 days, or refrigerate for up to 5 days.

Double-Chocolate Zucchini Bread

MAKES 1 (9-BY-5-INCH) LOAF

Prep time: 25 minutes

Cook time: 50 minutes

Ingredients:

- Gluten-free cooking spray
- 225 grams grated zucchini
- 125 grams All-Purpose Flour Blend
- 50 grams all-natural unsweetened cocoa powder (not Dutch-process)
- 1 teaspoon xanthan gum
- ¾ teaspoon baking soda
- ¼ teaspoon baking powder
- ¼ teaspoon salt
- ½ teaspoon ground espresso
- 135 grams chocolate chips or nondairy alternative
- 100 grams cane sugar or granulated sugar
- 2 large eggs

- ¼ cup avocado oil or canola oil
- 60 grams vanilla Greek yogurt or nondairy alternative
- 1 teaspoon vanilla extract

Directions:

Step 1

Preheat the oven to 350°F. Coat a 9-by-5-inch loaf pan with cooking spray or line it with parchment paper.

Step 2

Place the zucchini between 2 paper towels to absorb most of the moisture.

Step 3

In a medium bowl, whisk the flour, cocoa powder, xanthan gum, baking soda, baking powder, salt, espresso, and chocolate chips.

Step 4

In a small bowl, whisk the sugar, eggs, oil, yogurt, and vanilla. Using a spatula, add the flour mixture and mix until combined. Do not overmix. Fold in the zucchini. Pour this thick batter into the prepared loaf pan.

Step 5

Bake for 45 to 50 minutes, or until a toothpick inserted into the center of the loaf comes out clean. This bread could take a little longer to cook.

Step 6

Let the bread cool in the pan for at least 15 minutes. Gently remove from the pan and transfer the bread to a wire rack to cool completely. Store leftovers in an airtight container at room temperature for up to 5 days, or freeze to enjoy a slice whenever you desire. Let each slice thaw naturally.

Chocolate Chip Banana Bread

MAKES 1 (9-BY-5-INCH) LOAF

Prep time: 15 minutes

Cook time: about 1 hour

Ingredients:

- Shortening or gluten-free cooking spray, for preparing the pan
- 250 grams All-Purpose Flour Blend
- 1 teaspoon ground cinnamon
- 1 teaspoon xanthan gum
- 1 teaspoon baking powder
- ½ teaspoon baking soda
- ¼ teaspoon salt
- 8 tablespoons (1 stick) butter or nondairy alternative
- 150 grams light brown sugar
- 2 large eggs
- 80 grams plain Greek yogurt or nondairy alternative
- 450 grams mashed bananas (about 4 large bananas)
- 1 teaspoon vanilla extract
- 90 grams mini semisweet chocolate chips or nondairy alternative

Directions:

Step 1

Preheat the oven to 350°F. Grease a 9-by-5-inch loaf pan with shortening or gluten-free cooking spray.

Step 2

In a medium bowl, whisk the flour, cinnamon, xanthan gum, baking powder, baking soda, and salt to combine.

Step 3

In a large bowl, using a handheld electric mixer on medium speed, cream together the butter and brown sugar. Add the eggs and mix well, stopping to scrape down the bowl, as needed. Add the yogurt, bananas, and vanilla and mix well.

Step 4

Add half the flour mixture, reduce the mixer speed, and mix to combine. Add the remaining flour mixture and mix just until the batter is combined. Do not overmix. Using a rubber spatula, fold in the chocolate chips. Pour the batter into the prepared loaf pan.

Step 5

Bake for 1 hour, or until a toothpick inserted into the center of the bread comes out clean.

Step 6

Let the bread cool in the pan for at least 20 minutes, then gently transfer it to a wire rack to cool completely.

Apple Cinnamon Muffins

MAKES 12 MUFFINS

Prep time: 15 minutes
Cook time: 25 minutes

Ingredients:

- 250 grams All-Purpose Flour Blend
- 3 teaspoons ground cinnamon, divided
- 2 teaspoons baking powder
- 1 teaspoon baking soda
- 1 teaspoon xanthan gum
- ½ teaspoon salt
- ½ teaspoon gluten-free apple pie spice
- 80 grams unsweetened applesauce
- ½ cup avocado oil or canola oil
- ½ cup maple syrup
- 2 large eggs
- 2 teaspoons vanilla extract
- 240 grams grated Granny Smith or Honeycrisp apple
- 1 tablespoon cane sugar or granulated sugar

Directions:

Step 1

Preheat the oven to 425°F. Line a 12-cup muffin tin with cupcake liners.

Step 2

In a medium bowl, whisk the flour, 2 teaspoons of cinnamon, the baking powder, baking soda, xanthan gum, salt, and apple pie spice to blend.

Step 3

In a large bowl, whisk the applesauce, oil, maple syrup, eggs, and vanilla until blended.

Step 4

Using a rubber spatula, blend half the flour mixture into the applesauce mixture to incorporate. Add the remaining flour mixture, folding until just combined. Do not overmix. Fold in the apple. Evenly divide the batter between the prepared muffin cups.

Step 5

In a small bowl, mix the sugar and remaining 1 teaspoon of cinnamon. Generously sprinkle the cinnamon sugar over each muffin.

Step 6

Bake for 5 minutes to let the muffins set, then (without opening the oven) reduce the oven temperature to 350°F and bake for 20 minutes more, or until a toothpick inserted into the center of a muffin comes out clean.

Step 7

Let the muffins cool in the pan for 10 minutes, then transfer them to a wire rack to cool completely. Store leftovers in an airtight container for about 3 days at room temperature, or refrigerate for up to 5 days.

Coffee Cake Muffins

MAKES 12 MUFFINS

Prep time: 15 minutes

Cook time: 25 minutes

Ingredients:

FOR THE TOPPING

- 4 tablespoons butter or nondairy alternative
- 125 grams All-Purpose Flour Blend
- ¼ teaspoon xanthan gum
- 50 grams cane sugar or granulated sugar
- 50 grams light brown sugar
- 1 teaspoon ground cinnamon
- ¼ teaspoon salt

FOR THE MUFFINS

- 250 grams All-Purpose Flour Blend
- 2 teaspoons baking powder
- 1 teaspoon xanthan gum
- 1 teaspoon ground cinnamon
- ½ teaspoon baking soda
- ¼ teaspoon salt
- 100 grams light brown sugar
- ¾ cup whole milk or coconut milk beverage
- ⅓ cup avocado oil or canola oil
- 2 large eggs
- 2 teaspoons vanilla extract

FOR THE GLAZE

- 30 grams powdered sugar

- 1 teaspoon whole milk or coconut milk beverage
- ½ teaspoon vanilla extract

Directions:

Step 1

Preheat the oven to 425°F. Line a 12-cup muffin tin with cupcake liners.

TO MAKE THE TOPPING

Step 2

In a small saucepan, melt the butter over low heat. Set aside to cool.

Step 3

In a small bowl, whisk the flour and xanthan gum to blend. Add the cane sugar, brown sugar, cinnamon, and salt. Slowly pour in the melted butter, whisking. Do not use a spatula (which would make the mixture creamy); the whisk will separate the ingredients to produce a crumb consistency. Spread the topping on a piece of parchment paper to dry.

TO MAKE THE MUFFINS

Step 4

In a medium bowl, whisk the flour, baking powder, xanthan gum, cinnamon, baking soda, salt, and brown sugar to combine.

Step 5

In a large bowl, using a whisk or handheld electric mixer on medium speed, combine the milk, oil, eggs, and vanilla.

Step 6

Add half of the flour mixture to the milk mixture, mix them on low speed, then add the remaining half of the flour mixture and mix just until a batter is formed. Do not overmix. Evenly divide the batter between the prepared muffin cups.

Step 7

Generously sprinkle each muffin with the topping and gently pat it down with your fingertips.

Step 8

Bake for 5 minutes to let the muffins set, then (without opening the oven) reduce the oven temperature to 350°F and bake for 20 minutes more, or until a toothpick inserted into the center of a muffin comes out clean.

Step 9

Let the muffins cool in the pan for 10 minutes, then transfer them to a wire rack to cool completely.

TO MAKE THE GLAZE

Step 10

While the muffins cool, in a small bowl, whisk the powdered sugar, milk, and vanilla until smooth.

Step 11

Drizzle the glaze over each cooled muffin. Store leftover muffins in an airtight container for about 3 days at room temperature, or refrigerate for up to 5 days.

Veggie Muffins

MAKES 12 MUFFINS
Prep time: 30 minutes
Cook time: 25 minutes

Ingredients:

- 150 grams grated zucchini (about 2 small zucchini)
- 250 grams All-Purpose Flour Blend
- 2 teaspoons ground cinnamon
- 2 teaspoons baking powder
- 1 teaspoon xanthan gum
- ½ teaspoon baking soda
- ½ teaspoon salt
- ¼ teaspoon ground nutmeg
- 100 grams cane sugar or granulated sugar
- ½ cup avocado oil or canola oil
- 2 large eggs
- 2 teaspoons vanilla extract
- 55 grams grated carrot (about 2 carrots)

Directions:

Step 1

Preheat the oven to 425°F. Line a 12-cup muffin tin with cupcake liners.

Step 2

Place the grated zucchini between 2 paper towels to absorb most of the moisture.

Step 3

In a medium bowl, whisk the flour, cinnamon, baking powder, xanthan gum, baking soda, salt, and nutmeg to combine.

Step 4

In a small bowl, whisk the sugar, oil, eggs, and vanilla to blend. Using a spatula, add the flour mixture and mix until combined. Do not overmix. Using a spatula, fold in the zucchini and carrots. Evenly divide the batter between the prepared muffin cups.

Step 5

Bake for 5 minutes to let the muffins set, then (without opening the oven) reduce the oven temperature to 350°F and bake for 20 minutes, or until a toothpick inserted into the center of a muffin comes out clean.

Step 6

Let the muffins cool in the pan for 10 minutes, then transfer them to a wire rack to cool completely. Serve warm or cool. Keep covered at room temperature for up to 3 days or refrigerate for up to 5 days. You can also freeze them in a freezer bag. Let them thaw naturally or place in a 350°F oven for 5 to 7 minutes to warm.

Easy Drop Biscuits

MAKES 12 BISCUITS

Prep time: 15 minutes
 Cook time: 15 minutes

Ingredients:

- Shortening, for preparing the pan
- 375 grams All-Purpose Flour Blend
- 2 tablespoons baking powder

- 2 teaspoons cane sugar or granulated sugar
- 1½ teaspoons xanthan gum
- ½ teaspoon salt
- 6 tablespoons cold butter, divided
- 102 grams shortening
- 1 large egg
- 1 tablespoon honey, plus 2 teaspoons
- 1½ cups buttermilk, or 1½ cups coconut milk beverage plus 1½ tablespoons apple cider vinegar (see here)

Directions:

Step 1

Preheat the oven to 425°F. Grease a 12-cup muffin-top pan (yes, a pan that just makes muffin tops) with a light coating of shortening. (Or line a baking sheet with parchment paper.)

Step 2

In the bowl of a food processor, combine the flour, baking powder, sugar, xanthan gum, and salt and pulse about 5 times. Cut 4 tablespoons of butter into small pieces and add it to the food processor. Add the shortening in 3 portions, pulsing after each addition until a sand-like consistency forms.

Step 3

Add the egg, 2 teaspoons of honey, and ¾ cup of buttermilk. As you pulse the machine, drizzle the remaining ¾ cup of buttermilk through the feed tube. Keep pulsing until a thick batter forms. You may want to give it a stir to make sure the bottom ingredients are completely mixed in.

Step 4

Using a 2-tablespoon ice cream scoop, portion the batter into the prepared muffin-top cups. (Or place them about 2 inches apart on the lined baking sheet.)

Step 5

Bake for 13 to 15 minutes, or until the edges begin to brown.

Step 6

While the biscuits bake, in a small saucepan, melt the remaining 2 tablespoons of butter and 1 tablespoon of honey over medium-low heat.

Step 7

As soon as the biscuits come out of the oven, using a pastry brush, brush them with the honey-butter topping. Serve warm. These biscuits are best served same day, but you can refrigerate leftovers in an airtight container for up to 3 days, or freeze for up to 1 month. Warm in a 350°F oven for 5 to 7 minutes.

Garlic and Herb Drop Biscuits

MAKES 12 BISCUITS

Prep time: 15 minutes
Cook time: 25 minutes

Ingredients:

- Shortening for preparing the pan
- 6 tablespoons cold butter or nondairy alternative, divided
- 2½ teaspoons garlic powder, divided
- 375 grams All-Purpose Flour Blend

- 2 tablespoons baking powder
- 1½ teaspoons xanthan gum
- 1 teaspoon salt
- 1½ teaspoons dried oregano
- ½ teaspoon dried parsley
- ½ teaspoon dried thyme
- 6 to 8 fresh basil leaves, chopped
- 102 grams shortening
- 1 large egg
- 2 teaspoons honey
- 1½ cups buttermilk, or 1½ cups coconut milk beverage plus 1½ tablespoons apple cider vinegar (see here)

Directions:

Step 1

Preheat the oven to 425°F. Grease a 12-cup muffin-top pan (yes, a pan that just makes muffin tops) with shortening. (Or line a baking sheet with parchment paper.)

Step 2

In a small saucepan, melt 2 tablespoons of butter over low heat. Add 1 teaspoon of garlic powder. Bring the mixture to a boil and cook until the garlic is completely dissolved, about 3 minutes. Remove from the heat and set the garlic butter aside.

Step 3

In the bowl of a food processor, combine the flour, baking powder, xanthan gum, salt, remaining 1½ teaspoons of garlic powder, oregano, parsley, thyme, and basil and pulse about 5 times. Cut the remaining 4 tablespoons of butter into small pieces and add it to the food processor. Add the shortening in 3 portions, pulsing after each addition until a sand-like consistency forms.

Step 4

Add the egg, honey, and ¾ cup of buttermilk. As you pulse the machine, drizzle the remaining ¾ cup of buttermilk through the feed tube, pulsing until a thick batter forms. Give it a stir to make sure the bottom ingredients are completely mixed in.

Step 5

Using a 2-tablespoon ice cream scoop, portion the batter into the prepared muffin cups. (Or place them a few inches apart on the lined baking sheet.)

Step 6

Bake for 13 minutes. Remove from the oven and, using a pastry brush, immediately brush with some of the garlic butter. Bake for 3 to 5 minutes more, or until the edges begin to brown.

Step 7

Immediately remove and brush the biscuits again with the remaining garlic butter. Serve warm. Refrigerate leftovers in an airtight container for up to 3 days, or freeze for up to 1 month. Warm in a 350°F oven for 5 to 7 minutes.

Classic Biscuits

MAKES 6 BISCUITS
Prep time: 45 minutes
Cook time: 15 minutes

Ingredients:

- 136 grams shortening
- 312 grams All-Purpose Flour Blend , plus more for dusting
- 2 tablespoons baking powder
- 1 teaspoon xanthan gum
- 1 teaspoon baking soda
- 1 teaspoon salt
- 2 teaspoons cane sugar or granulated sugar
- 1 large egg
- 1 cup buttermilk, or 1 cup coconut milk beverage plus 1 tablespoon apple cider vinegar (see here), chilled, divided
- 2 tablespoons butter or nondairy alternative
- 1 tablespoon honey

Directions:

Step 1

Place the shortening in a small bowl and freeze for at least 30 minutes.

Step 2

Preheat the oven to 475°F. For best results, use a well-seasoned cast-iron skillet. (Or line a baking sheet with parchment paper.)

Step 3

In a medium bowl, whisk the flour, baking powder, xanthan gum, baking soda, salt, and sugar to combine. Add the cold shortening and use a pastry cutter to cut it into the flour mixture until you have a very coarse crumb.

Step 4

Place two sheets of parchment paper on a work surface and dust them well with flour.

Step 5

Make a well in the center of the flour mixture and add the egg and ¾ cup of chilled buttermilk. Using a spatula, fold the dough together. The less you touch the dough by hand, the better. The dough will seem crumbly; that's okay. Transfer the dough to the floured work surface. Pat the dough into a rectangle about 1 inch thick.

Step 6

Fold the dough into thirds, bringing in the left and right sides. This is called laminating the dough to produce layers. Next, fold in the top and bottom sides. Repeat this process one more time. Shape the dough into one last rectangle, about 6 by 9 inches and 1 inch thick.

Step 7

Place the second piece of parchment on top of the biscuit dough and gently smooth the top using a rolling pin, without flattening the rectangle. Using a 3-inch square cutter, cut out 6 biscuits. The biscuits are square so they touch and stick to each other to help them expand and rise. Rounds will not give you the same results. Transfer the biscuits to the skillet, placing them so they touch.

Step 8

Using a pastry brush, brush the tops with a light coating of the remaining buttermilk (you might not use all of it).

Step 9

Bake for 15 minutes, or until the biscuits turn lightly golden.

Step 10

While the biscuits bake, in a small saucepan, combine the butter and honey and melt over medium-low heat.

Step 11

Brush the honey butter over the biscuits as soon as they come out of the oven. They are best served warm the same day, with jam, butter, or bacon. They can also be frozen in a freezer bag for up to 1 month.

Toasted Coconut Apple Raspberry Crisp

MAKES 1 (9-BY-9-INCH) CRISP

Prep time: 20 minutes
Cook time: 37 minutes

Ingredients:

FOR THE TOASTED COCONUT

- 50 grams shredded coconut

FOR THE FILLING

- Shortening, for preparing the pan
- 2 Granny Smith or Honeycrisp apples, peeled and very thinly sliced
- 62 grams raspberries
- 1 tablespoon fresh lemon juice
- 1 teaspoon ground cinnamon

FOR THE OAT TOPPING

- 50 grams certified gluten-free rolled oats
- 2 tablespoons All-Purpose Flour Blend
- 2 tablespoons light brown sugar
- ¼ teaspoon xanthan gum
- 1 tablespoon maple syrup
- 2 tablespoons butter or nondairy alternative

Directions:

TO TOAST THE COCONUT

Step 1

Preheat the oven to 325°F. Line a baking sheet with parchment paper.

Step 2

Spread the coconut into a thin layer on the parchment and toast for 5 to 7 minutes until golden. Set aside.

Step 3

Leave the oven on and increase the temperature to 350°F.

TO MAKE THE FILLING

Step 4

Grease a 9-by-9-inch pan with shortening.

Step 5

In a medium bowl, combine the apples, raspberries, lemon juice, and cinnamon. Using a spatula, fold together the fruit and spread it in the prepared pan.

TO MAKE THE OAT TOPPING

Step 6

In a small bowl, whisk the oats, flour, brown sugar, and xanthan gum to combine. Add the maple syrup and butter. Using a pastry cutter, cut the butter into the mixture until crumbs form.

Step 7

Sprinkle the topping evenly over the fruit.

Step 8

Bake for 25 to 30 minutes, or until the topping is golden brown.

Step 9

Let the crisp cool for about 10 minutes. Sprinkle the toasted coconut over the top and serve. Refrigerate leftovers, covered, for up to 3 days.

Strawberry Streusel Crisp

MAKES 1 (11-BY-7-INCH) CRISP

Prep time: 15 minutes
Cook time: 45 minutes

Ingredients:

Shortening, for preparing the pan

FOR THE FILLING

- 100 grams cane sugar or granulated sugar
- 32 grams All-Purpose Flour Blend
- ¼ teaspoon xanthan gum
- ¼ teaspoon salt
- 800 grams sliced strawberries
- 1 tablespoon vanilla extract

FOR THE STREUSEL TOPPING

- 133 grams light brown sugar
- 85 grams All-Purpose Flour Blend
- 1 teaspoon ground cinnamon
- ¼ teaspoon xanthan gum
- ¼ teaspoon salt
- 8 tablespoons (1 stick) cold butter or nondairy alternative
- 66 grams gluten-free certified oats

Directions:

Step 1

Preheat the oven to 350°F. Grease an 11-by-7-inch pan with shortening.

TO MAKE THE FILLING

Step 2

In a large bowl, whisk the cane sugar, flour, xanthan gum, and salt to combine. Add the strawberries and vanilla. Using a spatula, gently toss everything together.

Step 3

Pour the strawberry mixture into the prepared baking dish and refrigerate until needed.

TO MAKE THE STREUSEL TOPPING

Step 4

In a medium bowl, whisk the brown sugar, flour, cinnamon, xanthan gum, and salt to combine. Smooth any clumps of brown sugar.

Step 5

Cut the butter into pieces and add it to the flour mixture. Using a pastry cutter, cut the butter into the flour mixture until crumbs form. Using a spatula, fold in the oats.

Step 6

Remove the filling from the refrigerator and cover it evenly with the topping.

Step 7

Bake for 40 to 45 minutes, or until the topping is crisp and the filling is bubbling.

Step 8

Let the streusel crisp cool on a wire rack for about 10 minutes. Serve warm or cooled. Refrigerate leftovers, covered, for up to 3 days.

Angel Food Cake

MAKES 1 (10-INCH) CAKE
Prep time: 25 minutes
Cook time: about 1 hour

Ingredients:

- 156 grams All-Purpose Flour Blend
- 350 grams cane sugar or granulated sugar
- 2 tablespoons arrowroot
- ½ teaspoon xanthan gum
- ¼ teaspoon salt
- 1½ cups egg whites (about 12 large eggs; see Tip)
- 1 teaspoon cream of tartar
- ½ teaspoon vanilla extract
- ½ teaspoon orange extract

Directions:

Step 1

Position an oven rack to the third lowest position and preheat the oven to 325°F.

Step 2

In a food processor, combine the flour, sugar, arrowroot, xanthan gum, and salt. Process to a fine powdery texture.

Step 3

In a large bowl, using a handheld electric mixer, beat the egg whites until they form stiff peaks. Be careful not to overmix. Add the cream of tartar, vanilla, and orange extract and give a quick stir with a spatula.

Step 4

Using the spatula, fold the flour mixture into the egg whites. Do not overmix.

Step 5

Pour the batter into an ungreased 10-inch tube pan.

Step 6

Bake for 50 to 60 minutes, or until a toothpick inserted into the center of the cake comes out clean.

Step 7

On a wire rack, invert the cake and let it cool in the pan. When completely cooled, remove the cake from the pan. Keep leftovers covered at room temperature for up to 3 days, or refrigerate for up to 5 days.

Carrot Cake

MAKES 1 (9-INCH) TWO-LAYER FROSTED CAKE

Prep time: 30 minutes

Cook time: about 35 minutes

Ingredients:

FOR THE CAKE

- Shortening, for preparing the pan
- 250 grams All-Purpose Flour Blend , plus more for dusting
- 62 grams arrowroot
- 2 teaspoons baking powder
- 2 teaspoons ground cinnamon
- 1 teaspoon xanthan gum
- 1 teaspoon baking soda
- 1 teaspoon ground ginger
- ½ teaspoon salt
- ¼ teaspoon ground nutmeg
- ¼ teaspoon ground cloves
- 300 grams light brown sugar
- 100 grams cane sugar or granulated sugar
- 1 cup avocado oil or canola oil
- 4 large eggs
- 180 grams unsweetened applesauce
- 1 teaspoon vanilla extract
- 1 teaspoon apple cider vinegar
- 220 grams grated carrot (about 6 small carrots)
- 55 grams canned crushed pineapple, drained (optional)
- 50 grams shredded coconut (optional)
- 62 grams chopped nuts (optional)

FOR THE CREAM CHEESE FROSTING

- 2 (8-ounce) packages cream cheese or nondairy alternative
- 8 tablespoons (1 stick) butter or nondairy alternative
- 2 to 3 tablespoons whole milk or coconut milk beverage
- 1 teaspoon vanilla extract
- ⅛ teaspoon salt
- 720 grams powdered sugar

Directions:

TO MAKE THE CAKE

Step 1

Preheat the oven to 350°F. Grease two 9-inch springform pans with shortening. Sprinkle a little flour inside and tap the pans to spread the flour evenly around each pan.

Step 2

In a medium bowl, whisk the flour, arrowroot, baking powder, cinnamon, xanthan gum, baking soda, ginger, salt, nutmeg, and cloves to combine.

Step 3

In a large bowl, using a whisk or handheld electric mixer, beat together the brown sugar, cane sugar, oil, eggs, applesauce, vanilla, and vinegar until combined, making sure there are no clumps of brown sugar remaining.

Step 4

Using a spatula, fold the flour mixture into the wet ingredients in two parts, mixing between each. Fold until just combined. Gently fold in the carrots. If using, fold in the pineapple, coconut, and nuts.

Step 5

Evenly divide the batter between the prepared cake pans.

Step 6

Bake for 30 to 35 minutes, or until a toothpick inserted in the center of a cake comes out clean.

Step 7

Let the cakes cool in the pans for 15 minutes. Release the clamp from each pan and remove the sides. Transfer the cakes and plates to a wire rack to cool completely.

TO MAKE THE CREAM CHEESE FROSTING

Step 8

In a large bowl, using a handheld electric mixer on medium speed, cream together the cream cheese and butter until smooth.

Step 9

Reduce the speed to low and add the milk, vanilla, salt, and powdered sugar. Mix until smooth and creamy.

Step 10

Frost the cake as desired. Refrigerate leftovers, covered, for up to 4 days.

Gooey Butter Cake

MAKES 1 (9-BY-13-INCH) CAKE
Prep time: 15 minutes
Cook time: about 45 minutes

Ingredients:

FOR THE BOTTOM CAKE LAYER

- Shortening, for preparing the pan
- 250 grams All-Purpose Flour Blend
- 150 grams cane sugar or granulated sugar
- 1 tablespoon baking powder
- 1 teaspoon xanthan gum
- 8 tablespoons (1 stick) butter or nondairy alternative, melted
- 2 large eggs
- 1 teaspoon vanilla extract

FOR THE TOP CREAMY LAYER

- 1 (8-ounce) package cream cheese or nondairy alternative
- 2 large eggs
- 1 teaspoon vanilla extract

- 480 grams powdered sugar

Directions:
TO MAKE THE BOTTOM CAKE LAYER

Step 1

Preheat the oven to 350°F. Grease a 9-by-13-inch pan with shortening.

Step 2

In a medium bowl, whisk the flour, sugar, baking powder, and xanthan gum to combine. Add the melted butter, eggs, and vanilla. Using a spatula, stir to combine.

Step 3

Using your clean hands, continue to mix, forming a dough. Press it firmly into the prepared pan.

TO MAKE THE TOP CREAMY LAYER

Step 4

In a large bowl, using a handheld electric mixer, beat the cream cheese until smooth. Add the eggs and vanilla. Mix for 2 minutes until well combined.

Step 5

With the mixer on low speed, slowly add the powdered sugar, 120 grams (1 cup) at a time. Mix until a batter forms. Pour the batter over the bottom layer.

Step 6

Bake for 40 to 45 minutes, or until the top becomes golden.

Step 7

Let the cake cool before slicing. Refrigerate leftovers, covered, for up to 1 week.

Lemon Lover's Bundt Cake

MAKES 1 BUNDT CAKE
Prep time: 45 minutes
Cook time: 50 minutes

Ingredients:
FOR THE CAKE

- Shortening, for preparing the pan
- 375 grams All-Purpose Flour Blend
- 1 teaspoon xanthan gum
- 1 teaspoon salt
- ½ teaspoon baking powder
- ½ teaspoon baking soda
- 16 tablespoons (2 sticks) butter or nondairy alternative
- 400 grams cane sugar or granulated sugar
- 4 large eggs
- ½ teaspoon vanilla extract
- 30 grams grated lemon zest (about 8 lemons)
- ½ cup fresh lemon juice (about 4 lemons)
- 1 cup buttermilk, or 1 cup coconut milk beverage plus 1 tablespoon apple cider vinegar (see here)

FOR THE LEMON SYRUP

- 100 grams cane sugar or granulated sugar

- ½ cup fresh lemon juice (about 4 lemons)

FOR THE GLAZE

- 120 grams powdered sugar
- 2 tablespoons whole milk or coconut milk beverage
- ¼ teaspoon vanilla extract
- ¼ teaspoon lemon extract

Directions:

TO MAKE THE CAKE

Step 1

Preheat the oven to 350°F. Grease a 10- to 12-cup Bundt pan with shortening.

Step 2

In a medium bowl, whisk the flour, xanthan gum, salt, baking powder, and baking soda to combine.

Step 3

In a small bowl, using a handheld electric mixer on medium speed, cream together the butter and sugar.

Step 4

In a third bowl, whisk the eggs, vanilla, lemon zest, and lemon juice to blend. Add this to the creamed butter and sugar. Mix well to combine. It will look curdled, but that's okay.

Step 5

Add half the flour mixture and ½ cup of buttermilk to the egg mixture and mix on low speed to blend. Add the remaining ½ cup of buttermilk and then the remaining flour mixture and mix just until everything is combined. Do not overmix.

Step 6

Pour the batter into the prepared Bundt pan.

Step 7

Bake for 40 to 45 minutes, or until a toothpick inserted into the center of the cake comes out clean.

Step 8

Let the cake cool in the pan for 15 minutes while you prepare the lemon syrup.

TO MAKE THE LEMON SYRUP

Step 9

In a small saucepan, combine the sugar and lemon juice. Cook over medium heat, stirring, until the sugar is completely dissolved. Bring the syrup to a boil and boil for 2 to 3 minutes. Remove from the heat and let the syrup cool. It will thicken a little as it cools.

Step 10

Line a baking sheet with parchment paper and set a wire rack in the pan. Remove the cake from the Bundt pan and flip it over onto the wire rack. Slowly pour the cooled syrup over the cake and allow the cake to soak it up.

Step 11

Let the cake cool completely.

TO MAKE THE GLAZE

Step 12

In a small bowl, whisk the powdered sugar, milk, vanilla, and lemon extract until smooth. Drizzle the glaze over the cake top and serve.

Step 13

Keep covered at room temperature, or refrigerate, for up to 5 days.

Lemon Crème Brûlée Pie

MAKES 1 (9-INCH) PIE

Prep time: 25 minutes

Cook time: 45 minutes

FOR THE CRUST

Shortening, for preparing the pie plate

Homemade Graham Crackers

67 grams cane sugar or granulated sugar

8 tablespoons (1 stick) butter or nondairy alternative, melted

FOR THE FILLING

125 grams All-Purpose Flour Blend

½ teaspoon xanthan gum

3 tablespoons cane sugar or granulated sugar, divided

1 (14-ounce) can sweetened condensed whole milk or sweetened condensed coconut milk

6 large egg yolks

2 tablespoons whole milk or coconut milk beverage

2 tablespoons grated lemon zest (about 2 lemons)

⅓ cup fresh lemon juice (about 2 lemons)

Directions:

TO MAKE THE CRUST

Step 1

Preheat the oven to 350°F. Grease a 9-inch pie plate with shortening.

Step 2

Make the full recipe of graham crackers and save half for another use. You only need half the crackers to make the crumbs here. In a food processor, pulse the graham crackers into crumbs. Weigh out 210 grams of crumbs and place them in a large bowl. Add the sugar and melted butter and stir until the crumbs are well coated. Transfer the coated crumbs to the pie plate and press them into a thin layer along the bottom and up the sides as high as they will go, working from the middle of the pan toward the edges.

Step 3

Place a piece of parchment paper over the crust and, using the back of a spoon or bottom of a glass, press the crumbs firmly into the pie plate.

Step 4

Remove the parchment and bake for 10 minutes.

Step 5

Let the crust cool as you prepare the filling.

TO MAKE THE FILLING

Step 6

In a small bowl, whisk the flour, xanthan gum, and 1 tablespoon of sugar to combine.

Step 7

In a large bowl, whisk the condensed milk, egg yolks, and whole milk until smooth and creamy. Add the lemon zest and lemon juice and whisk until smooth. Add the flour mixture and continue to whisk until a smooth batter forms. Set aside for 3 minutes to thicken.

Step 8

Pour as much filling as possible into the crust without overfilling it. There will be some left over.

Step 9

Carefully transfer the pie to the oven and bake for 25 to 30 minutes, or until the center is set and doesn't jiggle.

Step 10

Let the pie cool to room temperature, then refrigerate.

Step 11

When ready to serve, preheat the broiler.

Step 12

Sprinkle the pie with the remaining 2 tablespoons of sugar.

Step 13

Broil for about 5 minutes, or until the sugar melts and the edges begin to brown, watching carefully to prevent burning.

Step 14

Cool for 1 to 2 minutes before serving. Refrigerate leftovers, covered, for up to 2 days.

Éclair Pie

MAKES 1 (9-INCH) PIE

Prep time: 20 minutes

Cook time: 8 minutes, plus 1 hour to chill

Ingredients:

FOR THE CRUST

- Shortening, for preparing the pan
- 1 single Perfect Piecrust

FOR THE FILLING

- 1 (8-ounce) package cream cheese or nondairy alternative
- 3 egg yolks, beaten
- 1 teaspoon vanilla extract
- 32 grams All-Purpose Flour Blend
- ¼ teaspoon xanthan gum
- ¼ teaspoon salt
- 1¾ cups heavy cream or 1 (14-ounce) can coconut cream
- 200 grams cane sugar or granulated sugar
- 1 (8-ounce) container whipped topping
- ½ cup chocolate chips or nondairy alternative, melted

Directions:

TO MAKE THE CRUST

Step 1

Preheat the oven to 400°F. Grease a 9-inch pie plate with shortening.

Step 2

Roll out and fit the pie dough into the pie plate as directed. Line the piecrust with parchment paper and fill the bottom with dried beans or pie weights.

Step 3

Blind bake the crust for about 15 minutes, or until the edges are golden. Remove from the oven and remove the lining and weights. Prick holes all over the bottom of the crust with a fork. Return to the oven for 10 to 12 minutes, until the crust begins to brown. Let the crust cool completely as you prepare the filling.

TO MAKE THE FILLING

Step 4

In a large bowl, using an electric mixer on medium speed, beat the cream cheese until smooth and creamy. Set aside.

Step 5

In a small bowl, whisk the egg yolks and vanilla to combine. In a separate small bowl, whisk together the flour, xanthan gum, and salt.

Step 6

In a medium saucepan, whisk together the cream and sugar over medium heat. Bring it to a boil, whisking occasionally, for about 2 minutes, then remove from the heat.

Step 7

Whisk the flour mixture into the egg mixture. Then, whisking constantly, use a ladle to slowly add a small and steady stream of the warm cream mixture to the flour/egg mixture. Keep whisking so the egg yolks do not scramble. Repeat with one more ladle of cream mixture.

Step 8

Add the egg mixture back to the saucepan and set over medium heat. Stir occasionally, until just a few bubbles begin to appear. Do not bring it to a full boil. Remove it from the heat again.

Step 9

Slowly add one ladle full of the egg mixture to the bowl of cream cheese and, using the electric mixer, mix on low speed. Adding the egg mixture too fast will cause the cream cheese to clump, so take your time. Once it is fully mixed in and creamy, repeat with another ladle of egg mixture. Then add the remaining mixture to form the pudding completely.

Step 10

Pour the filling into the baked piecrust and cover it tightly with plastic (the plastic should be touching the filling). Chill the pie for at least 3 hours or overnight for best results.

Step 11

Top the pie with a layer of whipped topping and drizzle the melted chocolate all over the top. Serve cold. Refrigerate leftovers, covered, for up to 3 days.

Baked Apple Cinnamon Hand Pies

MAKES 8 HAND PIES

Prep time: 25 minutes
Cook time: 20 minutes

Ingredients:

- Pastry Dough

- 100 grams light brown sugar
- 2 teaspoons ground cinnamon
- 9 grams <u>All-Purpose Flour Blend</u>, plus more for dusting
- 1 large egg
- 1 Honeycrisp apple, peeled and thinly sliced
- Glaze (from Cinnamon Roll Pancakes)
- Gluten-free apple pie spice, for garnish (optional)

Directions:

Step 1

Make the pastry dough as directed, divide into 4 portions, wrap in plastic wrap, and refrigerate.

Step 2

In a medium bowl, whisk the brown sugar, cinnamon, and flour to combine.

Step 3

Position an oven rack in the lower third of the oven and preheat the oven to 400°F. Line a baking sheet with parchment paper.

Step 4

Place two large sheets of parchment paper on a work surface and dust them with flour. Halve each dough portion so you have 8 small pieces of dough. Working with one piece at a time, roll the dough between the two sheets of parchment into an 8-by-5-inch rectangle about ⅛ inch thick. Using a bench scraper or pizza cutter, cut the rectangle in half to make 2 smaller rectangles, each measuring 4 by 5 inches.

Step 5

In a small bowl, whisk the egg with 1 tablespoon water to create an egg wash. Using a pastry brush, lightly brush the rectangles with the egg wash. Reserve the remaining egg wash.

Step 6

Sprinkle the brown sugar mixture onto half the rectangles, leaving about ¼-inch border. Place 4 or 5 apple slices on top of the brown sugar. Top each tart with one of the remaining dough rectangles, egg wash-side down. Gently seal the edges with your fingers, then use a fork to crimp them. Use a bench scraper to gently transfer the tarts to the prepared baking sheet. With a pastry brush, lightly brush each tart with the remaining egg wash. With a toothpick, make 8 holes on the top of each tart to vent steam.

Step 7

Bake for 20 minutes, or until golden brown.

Step 8

Cool on a wire rack for 5 to 10 minutes.

Step 9

Frost the cooled tarts with the glaze and sprinkle each with apple pie spice (if using). Keep leftovers in an airtight container at room temperature for up to 3 days.

Sweet Tart Cakelets

MAKES 6 (3-INCH) CAKELETS

Prep time: 50 minutes

Cook time: 18 minutes

Ingredients:

- Shortening, for preparing the molds

- 190 grams <u>All-Purpose Flour Blend</u>, plus more for dusting
- 2 tablespoons cane sugar or granulated sugar
- ½ teaspoon xanthan gum
- ¼ teaspoon salt
- 2 egg yolks
- 2 teaspoons vanilla extract
- 120 grams powdered sugar
- 6 tablespoons cold butter or nondairy alternative

Directions:

Step 1

Grease six 3-inch tart molds with removable bottoms with shortening. Place two sheets of parchment paper on a work surface and dust them with flour.

Step 2

In a medium bowl, whisk the flour, sugar, xanthan gum, and salt to combine.

Step 3

In a small bowl, using a fork, beat the eggs. Add the vanilla and powdered sugar and, using a wooden spoon, stir together, getting all the powdered sugar from the edges.

Step 4

Using a pastry cutter, cut the cold butter into the flour mixture until crumbs form. Add the egg mixture and stir with a spoon so your hands do not handle the dough too much, but use your hands as needed. The dough may seem dry and crumbly, but it comes together as you work the dough.

Step 5

Transfer the dough to the floured work surface and roll it between the two parchment sheets to about ¼ inch thick. Use a round cookie cutter slightly bigger than your tart pans to cut 6 rounds. Use a spatula if necessary to transfer the dough rounds into the tart pans and gently push them in and shape them. Prick the bottom of each with a fork. Refrigerate for at least 30 minutes.

Step 6

Preheat the oven to 350°F.

Step 7

Bake for 15 to 18 minutes, or until the edges are golden.

Step 8

Let the tarts cool in the pans for 10 to 15 minutes. Turn the pans upside-down to remove the tarts. Place them on a wire rack to cool completely before topping. Refrigerate, covered, for up to 1 week or freeze for up to 3 months.

Italian Cream Tarts (Pasticciotti)

MAKES 6 TARTS

Prep time: 2 hours 45 minutes
Cook time: 15 minutes

Ingredients:

FOR THE FILLING

- 32 grams All-Purpose Flour Blend
- ¼ teaspoon xanthan gum

- 4 large egg yolks
- 100 grams cane sugar or granulated sugar
- 1 teaspoon vanilla extract
- ¾ cup whole milk or coconut milk beverage
- ¾ cup heavy cream or nondairy alternative
- Grated zest of 1 lemon

FOR THE DOUGH

- 4 tablespoons butter or nondairy alternative
- 39 grams shortening
- 250 grams <u>All-Purpose Flour Blend</u>, plus more for dusting
- 1 teaspoon xanthan gum
- 100 grams cane sugar or granulated sugar
- 1 teaspoon baking powder
- ½ teaspoon salt
- 2 large eggs, divided
- ¼ cup whole milk or coconut milk beverage
- 1 teaspoon vanilla extract
- Powdered sugar, for dusting

Directions:

TO MAKE THE FILLING

Step 1

In a small bowl, whisk the flour and xanthan gum to combine.

Step 2

In a small bowl, whisk the egg yolks, cane sugar, and vanilla to blend.

Step 3

In a small saucepan, combine the milk, cream, and lemon zest. Heat over medium heat until hot but do not boil. Remove from the heat and cool for 5 minutes. Whisk in the egg and flour mixtures, mixing well until no clumps remain. Return the pan to medium heat. Cook, stirring constantly, for 5 to 7 minutes, or until thickened. Transfer to a glass bowl and cover with plastic wrap, pushing the plastic down so it touches the filling. Refrigerate for at least 1 hour or overnight.

TO MAKE THE DOUGH

Step 4

Place the butter and shortening in the freezer for 30 minutes.

Step 5

Place two sheets of parchment paper on a work surface and dust them with flour. Line a baking sheet with parchment or a silicone baking mat.

Step 6

In a small bowl, whisk the flour, xanthan gum, cane sugar, baking powder, and salt to combine. Using a pastry cutter, cut the chilled butter and shortening into the flour mixture until it forms crumbs. Add 1 egg, the milk, and vanilla. Using a spatula, stir to mix. Avoid touching the dough too much.

Step 7

Transfer the dough to the floured work surface and flatten it. Place a piece of parchment paper over the dough and roll it to ¼-inch thickness. Remove the top sheet of parchment and, using a 3-inch round cookie cutter, cut 6 rounds from the dough. Gently transfer them to the prepared baking sheet.

Step 8

Reroll the remaining dough and place the second sheet of parchment on top. Place the rolled dough, still between the parchment, on top of the cut-out rounds. Refrigerate for at least 15 minutes.

Step 9

In a small bowl, whisk the remaining egg and 1 tablespoon water to create an egg wash. Set aside.

Step 10

Remove all the dough from the refrigerator. Using the parchment, carefully transfer the rolled layer to a work surface. Uncover and let sit for 1 minute. Using the cookie cutter, cut out 6 more rounds.

Step 11

Using a 1-inch ice cream scoop, drop 1 or 2 scoops of filling on the first batch of rounds. Using a spatula, top the filling with a round from the second batch. Using your fingertip, rub some egg wash between the 2 dough layers of each tart. Save the remaining egg wash. Push down the edges of the top layer to seal with the bottom layer. If the dough cracks, smooth it with your finger. Refrigerate the sealed tarts for at least 1 hour.

Step 12

Preheat the oven to 425°F.

Step 13

Using a pastry brush, brush the egg wash over the top of each tart. Bake for 18 to 20 minutes, or until the edges are golden and the tops pick up a little color.

Step 14

Let the tarts cool for about 10 minutes on the baking sheet, then use a spatula to carefully transfer to a wire rack to cool completely. Once cooled, sift powdered sugar over the top. Refrigerate the tarts, covered, for up to 3 days.

Cinnamon Rolls

MAKES 12 CINNAMON ROLLS

Prep time: 1 hour 50 minutes
Cook time: 25 minutes

Ingredients:

FOR THE FILLING

- 8 tablespoons (1 stick) butter or nondairy alternative
- 150 grams light brown sugar
- 1 tablespoon ground cinnamon

FOR THE CINNAMON ROLLS

- Shortening, for preparing the pan
- 375 grams All-Purpose Flour Blend, plus more for dusting
- 1 teaspoon xanthan gum
- 1 teaspoon baking powder
- ½ teaspoon baking soda
- ½ teaspoon salt
- ½ cup whole milk or coconut milk beverage
- 67 grams cane sugar or granulated sugar
- 4 tablespoons butter or nondairy alternative
- 1 (7-gram) packet instant (fast-acting) yeast

- 1 large egg
- ½ teaspoon apple cider vinegar

FOR THE ICING
- 2 tablespoons butter or nondairy alternative
- 2 ounces cream cheese or nondairy alternative
- 1 teaspoon vanilla extract
- 120 grams powdered sugar

Directions:

Step 1

Preheat the oven to 200°F and, once it is preheated, turn it off. This creates a warm environment to help the dough rise later on.

TO MAKE THE FILLING

Step 2

In a large bowl, using a handheld electric mixer on medium speed, cream the butter until smooth and creamy.

Step 3

In a small bowl, whisk the brown sugar and cinnamon to blend. Add the cinnamon sugar to the butter and mix to form a paste.

TO MAKE THE CINNAMON ROLLS

Step 4

Lightly grease a 9-inch baking dish with shortening. Place two sheets of parchment paper on a work surface and dust them with flour.

Step 5

In a medium bowl, whisk the flour, xanthan gum, baking powder, baking soda, and salt to combine.

Step 6

In a small bowl, stir together the milk and cane sugar.

Step 7

In a small saucepan, melt the butter over low heat. Add the milk mixture and bring the temperature to between 100°F and 110°F. Transfer to a large bowl and add the yeast. Give it a quick stir and let sit for 5 minutes.

Step 8

Stir in the egg and vinegar until combined. Using a handheld electric mixer fitted with the dough hook, mix the flour mixture into the wet ingredients, mixing until a dough forms.

Step 9

Transfer the dough to the floured parchment and flatten it by hand. Place the other sheet of parchment on top and roll the dough into a rectangle about ⅛ inch thick. Remove the top piece of parchment paper and evenly spread the brown sugar paste all over the dough. Starting on a long side, carefully roll the dough into a tight log. Smooth any cracks that might appear and give it a gentle roll to seal the seam.

Step 10

Using a very sharp knife, cut the log into 12 even pieces. Be careful not to smash the log with each cut. (You can also use unflavored unwaxed dental floss.) Place the rolls into the prepared pan, cut-side up and touching. Cover with plastic wrap, covering all the edges. Place a piece of aluminum foil over the top. Place the pan in the warmed oven for 1 hour.

Step 11

Remove the pan from the oven and remove the plastic wrap. Re-cover the rolls with the foil.

Step 12

Preheat the oven to 375°F.

Step 13

Bake the rolls, covered, for 13 minutes. Remove the foil and bake for 12 minutes more, or until the filling is bubbling and rolls have picked up a little color.

TO MAKE THE ICING

Step 14

While the rolls bake, in a medium bowl, using a handheld electric mixer on medium speed, cream together the butter, cream cheese, and vanilla until smooth and creamy. Add the powdered sugar and mix until smooth.

Step 15

Using a pastry brush, cover the just-baked rolls with icing. Let set for 1 minute and cover again with any remaining icing. Keep leftovers covered at room temperature or in the refrigerator for up to 3 days.

Strawberry Shortcake Rolls

MAKES 12 ROLLS

Prep time: 1 hour 50 minutes
Cook time: 25 minutes

Ingredients:

FOR THE FILLING

- 1½ tablespoons All-Purpose Flour Blend
- ¼ teaspoon xanthan gum
- 332 grams sliced strawberries
- 2 tablespoons cane sugar or granulated sugar

FOR THE ROLLS

- Shortening, for preparing the pan
- 375 grams <u>All-Purpose Flour Blend</u>, plus more for dusting
- 1 teaspoon xanthan gum
- 1 teaspoon baking powder
- ½ teaspoon baking soda
- ½ teaspoon salt
- ½ cup whole milk or coconut milk beverage
- 67 grams cane sugar or granulated sugar
- 8 tablespoons butter or nondairy alternative, divided
- 1 (7-gram) packet instant (fast-acting) yeast
- 1 large egg
- ½ teaspoon apple cider vinegar

FOR THE TOPPING

- 1 cup chilled heavy cream or coconut cream
- 2 tablespoons powdered sugar

Directions:

Step 1

Preheat the oven to 200°F and, once it is preheated, turn it off. This creates a warm environment to help the dough rise later on.

TO MAKE THE FILLING

Step 2

In a small bowl, whisk the flour and xanthan gum to combine.

Step 3

In a saucepan, combine the strawberries and sugar and cook over medium heat for about 15 minutes, stirring occasionally, until the strawberries are coated and softened.

Step 4

Stir in the flour mixture to thicken the strawberries. Transfer to an airtight container and refrigerate for 30 minutes.

TO MAKE THE ROLLS

Step 5

Lightly grease a 9-inch baking dish with shortening. Place two sheets of parchment paper on a work surface and dust them with flour.

Step 6

In a medium bowl, whisk the flour, xanthan gum, baking powder, baking soda, and salt to combine.

Step 7

In a small bowl, stir together the milk and cane sugar.

Step 8

In a small saucepan, melt 4 tablespoons of the butter over low heat. Stir the milk mixture into the melted butter and bring the temperature to between 100°F and 110°F. Transfer to a large bowl and add the yeast. Give it a quick stir and let sit for 5 minutes.

Step 9

Stir in the egg and vinegar until combined. Using a handheld electric mixer fitted with the dough hook, mix the flour mixture into the wet ingredients, mixing until a dough forms.

Step 10

Transfer the dough to the floured parchment and flatten it by hand. Place the other sheet of parchment on top and roll the dough to about ⅛ inch thick. Remove the top piece of parchment and evenly spread the strawberry filling all over the dough. Cut the remaining butter into small pieces and scatter them over the strawberries. Starting on a long side, carefully roll the dough into a tight log. Smooth any cracks that might appear and give it a gentle roll to seal the seam.

Step 11

Using a very sharp knife, cut the log into 12 even pieces. Be careful not to smash the log with each cut. (You can also use unflavored unwaxed dental floss.) Place the rolls into the prepared pan, cut-side up and touching. Cover with plastic wrap, covering all the edges. Place a piece of aluminum foil over the top. Place the pan in the warmed oven for 1 hour.

Step 12

Remove the pan from the oven and remove the plastic wrap. Re-cover the rolls with the foil.

Step 13

Preheat the oven to 375°F.

Step 14

Bake the rolls, covered, for 13 minutes. Remove the foil and bake for 12 minutes more, or until the rolls have picked up a little color.

TO MAKE THE TOPPING

Step 15

Make sure the heavy cream is very cold. In a large bowl, using a handheld electric mixer, whip the chilled heavy cream and powdered sugar until smooth and fluffy.

Step 16

Let the rolls cool for about 15 minutes in the pan. Serve with a dollop of whipped cream. Refrigerate leftovers, covered, for up to 3 days.

Lemon Berry Turnovers

MAKES 8 TURNOVERS

Prep time: 30 minutes
Cook time: 30 minutes

Ingredients:

FOR THE FILLING

- 22 grams All-Purpose Flour Blend
- ¼ teaspoon xanthan gum
- 300 grams blueberries
- 100 grams cane sugar or granulated sugar
- 1 teaspoon vanilla extract

FOR THE TURNOVERS

- All-Purpose Flour Blend , for dusting
- Pastry Dough , divided into 4 portions
- 1 large egg

FOR THE LEMON GLAZE

- 120 grams powdered sugar, plus more as needed
- 2 tablespoons fresh lemon juice, plus more as needed

Directions:

TO MAKE THE FILLING

Step 1

In a small saucepan, whisk the flour and xanthan gum to combine. Set the pan over medium heat and stir in the blueberries, 2 tablespoons water, the sugar, and vanilla. Cook, stirring constantly, for 5 minutes. Increase the heat slightly to get a slight boil and cook for 1 minute, stirring to prevent burning. Transfer the blueberry filling to a clean bowl and refrigerate for 15 minutes to thicken.

TO MAKE THE TURNOVERS

Step 2

Position an oven rack in the lower third of the oven and preheat the oven to 400°F. Line a baking sheet with parchment paper.

Step 3

Place two sheets of parchment paper on a work surface and dust them with flour. Working with 1 dough portion at a time, roll the dough between the 2 parchment sheets to ¼ to ⅛ inch. Roll it thin, but not so thin it will break. Using a bench scraper or pizza cutter, cut the flattened dough into 2 (5-inch) squares. Repeat with the remaining 3 dough portions. You should have 8 squares.

Step 4

Put about 2 tablespoons of filling in the middle of each square. Using your bench scraper, lift one corner of the pastry dough and fold it diagonally over to make a triangle. Gently press down on the ends to seal. It's okay if some berries leak out. Using the tines of a fork, crimp the edges. Transfer to the baking sheet.

Step 5

In a small bowl, whisk the egg and 1 tablespoon water to create an egg wash. Using a pastry brush, lightly brush each turnover with egg wash. Using a knife, make 2 small slits in each to vent steam.

Step 6

Bake for 20 minutes, or until golden brown.

Step 7

Let the turnovers cool for 10 minutes on the baking sheet.

TO MAKE THE LEMON GLAZE

Step 8

In a small bowl, stir together the powdered sugar and lemon juice until smooth and thin enough to drizzle. If it's too thick, add more lemon juice; if it's too thin, add more powdered sugar.

Step 9

Using a fork, drizzle the turnovers with the glaze. Keep leftovers covered at room temperature for up to 3 days.

PB&J Turnovers

MAKES 8 TURNOVERS
Prep time: 30 minutes
Cook time: 20 minutes

Ingredients:

FOR THE FILLING

- 22 grams All-Purpose Flour Blend , plus more for dusting
- ¼ teaspoon xanthan gum
- 345 grams blackberries
- 100 grams cane sugar or granulated sugar
- 1 teaspoon vanilla extract

FOR THE TURNOVERS

- Pastry Dough , divided into 4 portions
- 1 large egg

FOR THE TOPPING

- 45 grams creamy gluten-free peanut butter, melted
- 1 tablespoon avocado oil or canola oil

Directions:

TO MAKE THE FILLING

Step 1

In a small saucepan, whisk the flour and xanthan gum to combine. Set the pan over medium heat and stir in the blackberries, 2 tablespoons water, the sugar, and vanilla. Cook, stirring constantly, for 5 minutes. Increase the heat slightly to get a slight boil and cook for 1 minute, stirring to prevent burning. Transfer the blackberry filling to a clean bowl and refrigerate for 15 minutes to thicken.

TO MAKE THE TURNOVERS

Step 2

Position an oven rack in the lower third of the oven and preheat the oven to 400°F. Line a baking sheet with parchment paper.

Step 3

Place two sheets of parchment paper on a work surface and dust them with flour. Working with 1 dough portion at a time, roll the dough between the two parchment sheets to ¼ to ⅛ inch. Roll it thin, but not so thin it will break. Using a bench scraper or pizza cutter, cut the flattened dough into 2 (5-inch) squares. Repeat with the remaining 3 dough portions. You should have 8 squares.

Step 4

Put about 2 tablespoons of filling in the middle of each square. Using your bench scraper, lift one corner of the pastry dough and fold it diagonally over to make a triangle. Gently press down on the ends to seal. It's okay if some berries leak out. Using the tines of a fork, crimp the edges. Transfer to the baking sheet.

Step 5

In a small bowl, whisk the egg and 1 tablespoon water to create an egg wash. Using a pastry brush, lightly brush each turnover with egg wash. Using a knife, make 2 small slits in each to vent steam.

Step 6

Bake for 20 minutes, or until golden brown.

Step 7

Let the turnovers cool for 10 minutes on the baking sheet.

TO MAKE THE TOPPING

Step 8

In a small microwave-safe bowl, combine the peanut butter and oil. Microwave in 15-second intervals, giving it a good stir between each, until melted.

Step 9

Using a fork, drizzle the peanut butter over the turnovers. Keep leftovers covered at room temperature for up to 3 days.

Mini French Crullers

MAKES 20 SMALL CRULLERS

Prep time: 1 hour 20 minutes, plus 1 hour to set
Cook time: 30 minutes

Ingredients:

- 125 grams All-Purpose Flour Blend
- ½ teaspoon xanthan gum
- ½ teaspoon salt
- ¼ teaspoon ground cinnamon
- 8 tablespoons (1 stick) butter or nondairy alternative
- 2 large eggs
- Oil or shortening, for frying
- Glaze (from Cinnamon Roll Pancakes)

Directions:

Step 1

Line a baking sheet with parchment paper.

Step 2

In a small bowl, whisk the flour, xanthan gum, salt, and cinnamon to combine.

Step 3

In a small saucepan, combine the butter and 1 cup water and bring to a boil over medium-high heat. Once at a boil, stir in the flour mixture. Remove it from the heat and let the mixture cool for 5 minutes.

Step 4

One at a time, add the eggs, thoroughly stirring after each addition. The batter will become smooth.

Step 5

Fit a piping bag with a 1M star tip and fill it with the batter. Pipe about 20 circles 1 to 2 inches in diameter on the prepared baking sheet. Freeze for at least 1 hour.

Step 6

Pour about 3 inches of oil into a large, deep heavy-bottomed pot and heat to 350°F over medium heat.

Step 7

Place a paper towel on a wire rack and place the rack on a baking sheet.

Step 8

Carefully add the frozen crullers to the hot oil and fry for 2 to 3 minutes per side until golden. Using tongs, transfer to the prepared rack to drain.

Step 9

Dip and coat each cruller in the glaze almost immediately and let set for about 1 hour.

Step 10

These are best served the same day. Keep leftovers in an airtight container at room temperature for up to 2 days.

Butterhorns

MAKES 12 BUTTERHORNS

Prep time: about 30 minutes, plus 3 hours to chill
Cook time: 30 minutes

Ingredients:

FOR THE FILLING

- 50 grams light brown sugar
- 2 teaspoons ground cinnamon

FOR THE BUTTERHORNS

- 250 grams <u>All-Purpose Flour Blend</u> , plus more for dusting
- 1 teaspoon salt
- ½ teaspoon xanthan gum
- 24 tablespoons (3 sticks) cold butter or nondairy alternative
- ½ cup cold sour cream or nondairy alternative
- 1 large egg yolk
- Glaze (from Cinnamon Roll Pancakes)

Directions:

TO MAKE THE FILLING

Step 1

In a small bowl, stir together the brown sugar and cinnamon. Set aside.

TO MAKE THE BUTTERHORNS

Step 2

Place two sheets of parchment paper on a work surface and dust them with flour.

Step 3

In a medium bowl, whisk the flour, salt, and xanthan gum to combine.

Step 4

Cut the butter into pieces and add it to the flour mixture. Using a pastry cutter, cut the butter into the flour until crumbs form. Add the sour cream, egg yolk, and 1 tablespoon water. Mix to form the dough.

Step 5

Transfer the dough to the floured parchment paper. Top with the second sheet of parchment and use a rolling pin to flatten the dough to a round about ¼ inch thick. Transfer the dough, still covered, to a baking sheet. Refrigerate for 15 minutes.

Step 6

Remove the dough from the refrigerator and test it to make sure it is pliable. If too stiff, let sit for 1 minute to soften.

Step 7

Line another baking sheet with parchment paper.

Step 8

Using a bench scraper or pizza cutter, cut the dough, as you would cut a pizza, into 16 triangles. Using a bench scraper, gently pull the triangles away from each other and make sure they are not sticking to the parchment.

Step 9

Working one at a time, sprinkle some of the filling onto each and roll the dough from the wide end to the tip. Place the "horn" on the prepared baking sheet, seam-side down, and bend it into a slight crescent shape. Cover with plastic wrap and refrigerate for at least 2 hours.

Step 10

Preheat the oven to 375°F.

Step 11

Bake on the parchment-lined sheet for 25 to 30 minutes until the edges have slightly browned.

Step 12

Let the horns cool on the baking sheet for 10 minutes, then gently transfer to a wire rack set over a paper towel.

Step 13

Dip each warm cookie in the glaze and let set for at least 30 minutes. Keep leftovers in an airtight container at room temperature for up to 3 days.

Cream Puffs

MAKES 10 CREAM PUFFS
Prep time: 20 minutes
 Cook time: about 50 minutes

Ingredients:
FOR THE CREAM PUFFS
- 1 large egg
- Choux Pastry

FOR THE FILLING
- 1 cup cold heavy cream or coconut cream
- 2 tablespoons powdered sugar, plus more for dusting
- ½ teaspoon vanilla extract

Directions:
TO MAKE THE CREAM PUFFS

Step 1

Preheat the oven to 425°F. Line a baking sheet with parchment paper. Prepare a piping bag with a 1A tip and set aside.

Step 2

In a small bowl, whisk the egg and 1 tablespoon water to create an egg wash. Set aside.

Step 3

Fill the piping bag with the Choux Pastry and lay it flat.

Step 4

Using a pastry brush, brush the parchment on the prepared baking sheet with water. This will create humidity in the oven.

Step 5

Pipe the batter onto the wet parchment in 10 swirls, as you would frost a cupcake, about 2 inches wide and 3 inches apart so they do not touch when they "puff" in the oven. Use a wet fingertip to smooth the top of each. Brush each with egg wash.

Step 6

Bake for 25 minutes, then (without opening the oven) reduce the temperature to 350°F and bake for 20 to 22 minutes more, or until golden. Turn off the oven and keep them inside for 5 to 7 minutes. This will help prevent them from sinking.

Step 7

Remove and let the pastries cool on the baking sheet for 10 minutes, then gently transfer to a wire rack to cool completely.

TO MAKE THE FILLING

Step 8

Make sure the heavy cream is very cold before preparing the filling.

Step 9

In a large bowl, using a handheld electric mixer, whip the cold heavy cream, powdered sugar, and vanilla until thick and fluffy.

Step 10

Split the pastries horizontally and fill them with cream. Dust with powdered sugar and serve. Refrigerate leftovers, covered, for up to 3 days.

Homemade Graham Crackers

MAKES 15 CRACKERS

Prep time: 15 minutes
Cook time: 15 minutes

Ingredients:

- 250 grams <u>All-Purpose Flour Blend</u> , plus more for dusting
- 63 grams brown rice flour
- 1 tablespoon ground cinnamon
- 1 teaspoon baking powder
- ½ teaspoon baking soda
- ½ teaspoon xanthan gum
- ¼ teaspoon salt
- 50 grams light brown sugar
- ⅓ cup avocado oil or canola oil
- ⅓ cup maple syrup
- ¼ cup whole milk or coconut milk beverage
- 2 tablespoons honey
- 1 tablespoon vanilla extract

Directions:

Step 1

Preheat the oven to 350°F. Place two sheets of parchment paper on a work surface and dust them with the all-purpose flour.

Step 2

In a medium bowl, whisk the all-purpose flour, rice flour, cinnamon, baking powder, baking soda, xanthan gum, and salt to combine.

Step 3

In a large bowl, using a handheld electric mixer, beat the brown sugar, oil, maple syrup, milk, honey, and vanilla. Add the flour mixture and mix with a spatula until combined. The dough will be sticky.

Step 4

Transfer the dough to the flour-dusted parchment. Place the second sheet of parchment on top and roll the dough into a large round a little less than ¼ inch thick. Trim off the edges to form a perfect square. Gather up the scraps and repeat the procedure (although the squares will get ever smaller) until all the dough has been cut into cracker shapes.

Step 5

Using the parchment, transfer the dough to a baking sheet. Using a pizza cutter or bench scraper, cut the dough horizontally and vertically to create squares the size of graham crackers, cutting through the dough but leaving everything in place. Prick each cracker with a fork 4 times and score a faint line in the middle of each cracker where it can be snapped in half.

Step 6

Bake for 15 minutes. (Bake the crackers a few more minutes for a crispier cracker.)

Step 7

Let the crackers cool on the baking sheet before you cut them. Keep the crackers in an airtight container at room temperature for up to 1 week, or freeze for up to 1 month.

Pastry Dough

MAKES ENOUGH FOR 8 (5-INCH) PASTRIES

Prep time: about 2 hours

Ingredients:

- 292 grams All-Purpose Flour Blend , plus 32 grams
- 1 teaspoon xanthan gum
- 1 teaspoon salt
- 8 tablespoons (1 stick) butter or nondairy alternative, chilled
- 67 grams chilled shortening, frozen for 30 minutes
- ½ cup ice-cold water

Directions:

Step 1

Place a sheet of parchment paper on a work surface and dust it with flour (you won't use all 32 grams at once—start with a little and add more as needed).

Step 2

In a food processor, combine the remaining 292 grams of flour, the xanthan gum, and salt. Pulse 1 to 3 times.

Step 3

Cut the chilled butter into pieces and add it to the food processor along with the chilled shortening. Pulse about 10 times until the mixture looks sandy.

Step 4

Slowly add the ice-cold water, pulsing after each addition, until the dough comes together. Transfer the dough to the floured parchment. If the dough is too wet, using your hands, work in some of the remaining 32 grams of flour until soft and pliable.

Step 5

Use this dough in the pastry recipe of your choice and follow the baking instructions. Chill the dough for 30 minutes after you roll it into your desired shape before baking. If not using immediately, roll it into a disc about 1 inch thick, wrap the dough in plastic wrap, and refrigerate for up to 3 days.

Choux Pastry

MAKES ENOUGH FOR 10 CREAM PUFFS

Prep time: 15 minutes

Ingredients:

- 125 grams All-Purpose Flour Blend , plus more as needed
- ¼ teaspoon xanthan gum
- 8 tablespoons (1 stick) butter or nondairy alternative, cut into tablespoon chunks
- ½ cup whole milk or coconut milk beverage
- 1 tablespoon cane sugar or granulated sugar
- ¼ teaspoon salt
- 4 large eggs

Directions:

Step 1

In a small bowl, whisk the flour and xanthan gum to combine.

Step 2

In a small saucepan, combine the butter, milk, ½ cup water, the sugar, and salt. Set over medium heat and cook, stirring with a wooden spoon, until the butter and sugar melt. Increase the heat for about 2 minutes until steam rises. Reduce the heat, add the flour mixture, and stir with a wooden spoon until a shiny gel-like ball forms.

Step 3

Transfer the dough to a large bowl and let it cool for about 5 minutes.

Step 4

In a medium bowl, beat the eggs until smooth and combined.

Step 5

Pour one-quarter of the beaten eggs into the dough. Using a handheld electric mixer on low speed, beat for 15 to 20 seconds to combine. Add another one-quarter of the beaten eggs to the bowl and mix again to combine. Repeat until almost all of the eggs are added. Be careful that the batter does not become runny. The ideal batter is thick enough that it will not drip out of the piping bag, but not too thick. You may not use all the beaten eggs. If your batter is runny, add 1 tablespoon of the flour blend (there is no need for additional xanthan gum).

Step 6

Fill the piping bag with the batter and use according to the recipe.

Sandwich Bread

MAKES 1 (9-BY-5-INCH) LOAF
Prep time: 3 hours 20 minutes
Cook time: 30 minutes

Ingredients:

- Shortening, for preparing the pan
- 375 grams Bread Flour Blend
- 3 tablespoons cane sugar or granulated sugar
- 1 tablespoon xanthan gum
- 2 teaspoons baking powder
- 1 teaspoon salt
- ½ teaspoon baking soda
- 1 (7-gram) packet instant (fast-acting) yeast
- 4 large eggs, divided
- ¼ cup extra-virgin olive oil
- 1 tablespoon honey
- 2 teaspoons apple cider vinegar
- 1 cup warm (100° to 110°F) whole milk or coconut milk beverage

Directions:

Step 1

Position an oven rack in the third lowest position. Grease a 9-by-5-inch loaf pan with shortening or line it with parchment paper.

Step 2

In a medium bowl, whisk the flour, sugar, xanthan gum, baking powder, salt, baking soda, and yeast to combine.

Step 3

In a small bowl, beat 3 of the eggs, the oil, honey, and vinegar. Add the egg mixture to the flour mixture and, using a handheld electric mixer, beat together as you slowly add the warm milk. Mix for 1 or 2 minutes until combined.

Step 4

Transfer the dough to the prepared loaf pan and spread it evenly, smoothing the top. Loosely cover the pan with plastic wrap and let the dough rest for 1 hour. Remove the plastic wrap and let the dough rest for 2 hours more, until it doubles in size.

Step 5

Preheat the oven to 425°F.

Step 6

In a small bowl, whisk the remaining egg and 1 tablespoon water to create an egg wash. Using a pastry brush, gently brush the loaf with the egg wash.

Step 7

Bake for 28 to 30 minutes, or until the top is golden brown.

Step 8

If you did not use parchment to line the pan, let the loaf cool in the pan for about 1 hour, then remove it from the pan. Use a butter knife to pull the bread away from the edges. Transfer it to a wire rack and let the loaf cool completely. If you used parchment paper, lift the loaf out of the pan after 30 minutes and transfer it to the rack. Slice and serve. Keep leftovers in an airtight bag at room temperature for up to 3 days or refrigerate for up to 1 week.

Burger Buns

MAKES 4 BUNS

Prep time: 3 hours 20 minutes
Cook time: 15 minutes

Ingredients:

- 190 grams Bread Flour Blend , plus more for dusting
- 1½ tablespoons cane sugar or granulated sugar
- 2 teaspoons instant (fast-acting) yeast
- 1½ teaspoons xanthan gum
- 1 teaspoon baking powder
- ½ teaspoon salt
- ¼ teaspoon baking soda
- 2 large eggs, divided
- 4 tablespoons extra-virgin olive oil, divided
- 1½ teaspoons honey
- 1 teaspoon apple cider vinegar
- ½ cup warm (100° to 110°F) whole milk or coconut milk beverage

Directions:

Step 1

Line a baking sheet with a silicone baking mat or parchment paper. Place a sheet of parchment on a work surface and dust it with flour.

Step 2

In a medium bowl, whisk the flour, sugar, yeast, xanthan gum, baking powder, salt, and baking soda to combine.

Step 3

In a small bowl, beat 1 of the eggs, 3 tablespoons of oil, the honey, and vinegar. Add the egg mixture to the flour mixture and, using a handheld electric mixer, beat slowly as you add the warm milk, 1 to 2 minutes until combined. Transfer the dough to the floured parchment and divide it into 4 equal portions.

Step 4

Place the remaining 1 tablespoon of oil in a small dish. Coat your fingertips and palms in the oil. Roll each dough portion into a smooth ball and place on the prepared baking sheet, gently pressing down to create a bun shape. Smooth the top, if needed. Loosely cover with plastic wrap and let the dough rest at least 3 hours.

Step 5

Position an oven rack in the lower third of the oven and preheat the oven to 425°F.

Step 6

In a small bowl, whisk the remaining egg and 1 tablespoon of water to create an egg wash. Using a pastry brush, gently brush each bun with the egg wash.

Step 7

Bake for 15 minutes, or until the buns are golden brown.

Step 8

Let the buns cool on the baking sheet for at least 15 minutes before cutting them in half horizontally. Keep leftovers in an airtight container at room temperature for up to 3 days. Reheat to serve.

Artisan Loaves

MAKES 2 SMALL LOAVES
Prep time: 1 hour 15 minutes
Cook time: 35 minutes

Ingredients:

- 250 grams Bread Flour Blend
- 1 tablespoon light brown sugar
- 2 teaspoons xanthan gum
- 1 teaspoon baking powder
- 1 teaspoon salt
- ¾ cup warm (100° to 110°F) water
- 1 teaspoon cane sugar or granulated sugar
- 1 (7-gram) packet instant (fast-acting) yeast
- 1 large egg, beaten
- 1 tablespoon olive oil, plus more for the piping bag
- 1 tablespoon honey
- ½ teaspoon apple cider vinegar

Directions:

Step 1

Position an oven rack in the lower third of the oven. Line a baguette pan with parchment paper.

Step 2

In a medium bowl, whisk the flour, brown sugar, xanthan gum, baking powder, and salt to combine.

Step 3

In a large bowl, combine the water, cane sugar, and yeast. Let sit for 5 minutes.

Step 4

Add the beaten egg, oil, honey, and vinegar and stir until combined. Using a handheld electric mixer fitted with the paddle attachment, add half the flour mixture and mix on low speed to combine. Add the remaining flour mixture and mix to form a wet dough.

Step 5

Pour a bit of oil into a piping bag or plastic bag, and massage the bag to spread the oil. Oil your fingertips and transfer the dough to the bag. Cut the tip to 1½ inches. Pipe the dough into the prepared pan to form two long loaves about 8 inches long. Let the dough rest, uncovered, for at least 1 hour.

Step 6

Preheat the oven to 425°F.

Step 7

Bake for 30 to 35 minutes, or until golden brown. Let the loaves cool for about 10 minutes in the pan, then transfer to a wire rack to cool for 15 to 20 minutes before slicing. Keep leftovers in an airtight container for up to 3 days. Rewarm to serve.

Soft French Loaves

MAKES 2 LOAVES

Prep time: 1 hour 20 minutes
Cook time: 25 minutes

Ingredients:

- 375 grams All-Purpose Flour Blend , plus more for dusting
- 32 grams brown rice flour
- 1 tablespoon xanthan gum
- 1½ teaspoons baking powder
- 1 teaspoon salt
- 3 tablespoons golden flax meal
- 2 tablespoons cane sugar or granulated sugar
- 1 (7-gram) packet instant (fast-acting) yeast
- 1 tablespoon honey
- 1¼ cups warm (100° to 110°F) water
- 3 large eggs, beaten, plus 1 large egg
- ½ cup avocado oil or canola oil, plus more for the oil bath and piping bags
- 1 tablespoon apple cider vinegar

Directions:

Step 1

Line a twin baguette pan with parchment paper, or line a baking sheet with parchment or a silicone baking mat.

Step 2

In a medium bowl, whisk the all-purpose flour, rice flour, xanthan gum, baking powder, and salt to combine.

Step 3

In large bowl, combine the flax meal, sugar, yeast, honey, and ¾ cup of warm water. Give it a stir and let sit for 5 minutes.

Step 4

Add the 3 beaten eggs, ½ cup of oil, remaining ½ cup of warm water, and vinegar and mix until combined. Using a handheld electric mixer fitted with a paddle attachment, add half the flour mixture to the wet ingredients and mix on low speed to combine. Add the remaining flour mixture and mix to form a dough. This dough will be more like a batter.

Step 5

Add a bit of oil to 2 piping bags or plastic bags and massage the bags to coat with the oil. Pour about 1 tablespoon of oil into a small bowl. Dip your fingertips in the oil and divide the dough into 2 portions. Place each portion in one of the prepared bags and cut the tips about 1¼ inches wide. Fill each side of the prepared pan with the batter from one of the bags. Let the dough rest and rise for 1 hour.

Step 6

Preheat the oven to 425°F.

Step 7

In a small bowl, whisk the remaining egg with 1 tablespoon water to create an egg wash. Using a pastry brush, lightly brush the egg wash over the loaves.

Step 8

Bake for 25 minutes.

Step 9

Let the loaves cool in the pan for at least 15 minutes before serving. Keep leftovers in an airtight bag at room temperature for up to 5 days.

Pillowy Dinner Rolls

MAKES 8 ROLLS

Prep time: 2 hours 20 minutes

Cook time: 25 minutes

Ingredients:

FOR THE ROLLS

- Shortening, for preparing the baking dish
- 250 grams Bread Flour Blend , plus more for dusting
- 1½ teaspoons xanthan gum
- 1 teaspoon baking powder
- ½ teaspoon salt
- 50 grams cane sugar or granulated sugar
- 1 (7-gram) packet instant (fast-acting) yeast
- 2 tablespoons butter or nondairy alternative, melted
- ½ cup warm (100° to 110°F) whole milk or coconut milk beverage
- 1 large egg, beaten
- 2 tablespoons honey
- ½ teaspoon apple cider vinegar
- 1 tablespoon olive oil

FOR THE TOPPING

- 2 tablespoons butter or nondairy alternative, melted
- 1 tablespoon honey

Directions:

TO MAKE THE ROLLS

Step 1

Grease a 9-by-9-inch baking dish with shortening. Place a piece of parchment paper on a work surface and dust it with flour.

Step 2

In a medium bowl, whisk the flour, xanthan gum, baking powder, and salt to combine.

Step 3

In a large bowl, stir together the sugar, yeast, melted butter, and warm milk. Let sit for 5 minutes.

Step 4

Add the beaten egg, honey, and vinegar to the yeast mixture and mix to combine. Using a handheld electric mixer fitted with the dough hook, add half the flour mixture to the wet ingredients and mix on low speed. Add the remaining flour mixture and mix to form a dough.

Step 5

Oil your fingertips and transfer the dough to the floured work surface. Divide the dough into 6 to 8 equal portions and roll them into balls, smoothing the tops and making sure the seams are on the bottom. Place the dough balls in the prepared baking dish so they barely touch. Cover with plastic wrap and let the dough rest and rise for at least 2 hours.

TO MAKE THE TOPPING

Step 6

In a small bowl, stir together the melted butter and honey. Using a pastry brush, brush each roll with some of the honey butter. Reserve the remainder.

Step 7

Preheat the oven to 375°F.

Step 8

Bake the rolls for 22 to 25 minutes, or until slightly golden.

Step 9

Remove from the oven and brush the reserved honey butter over the top; they will begin to pick up more color. Let the rolls cool in the pan for about 10 minutes before serving warm with butter. Keep leftovers covered at room temperature for 1 day. Reheat before serving again.

Tortilla Wraps

MAKES 6 TO 8 TORTILLAS

Prep time: 15 minutes
Cook time: 30 to 40 minutes

Ingredients:

- 375 grams All-Purpose Flour Blend
- 3 tablespoons cane sugar or granulated sugar
- 2 teaspoons baking powder
- 1½ teaspoons xanthan gum
- 1 teaspoon salt
- 68 grams shortening
- 2 tablespoons avocado oil or canola oil
- ¾ cup plus 1 tablespoon cold water

Directions:

Step 1

In a medium bowl, whisk the flour, sugar, baking powder, xanthan gum, and salt to combine. Using your fingers, rub the shortening through the flour until crumbs form. Add the oil and ¾ cup of cold water. Using your hands, form the dough until it is very pliable, like cookie dough that can easily be rolled into a ball, adding up to 1 tablespoon of water as needed.

Step 2

Divide the dough into 6 to 8 portions, depending on the size of your tortilla press, and roll each into a ball.

Step 3

Preheat a nonstick skillet over medium heat.

Step 4

Cut two pieces of parchment paper to fit your tortilla press. Place one dough ball between the pieces of parchment and place it into the press. Press and flatten to about ⅛ inch.

Step 5

Open the press and remove the top piece of parchment. Gently pick up the tortilla with the bottom piece of parchment and flip it into the hot skillet. Cook the tortilla for 2 to 3 minutes, or until air bubbles appear and it easily slides in the skillet. Flip the tortilla and cook the other side for 1 to 2 minutes more, or until it slides easily. The second side will not take as long to cook, so watch it to prevent burning.

Step 6

When the tortilla is ready, transfer it to a plate. Gently fold the tortilla, but avoid making a crease in the center. Repeat with the remaining dough balls.

Printed in Great Britain
by Amazon